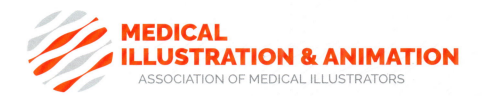

MEDILLSB.COM

34

EDITOR Rachel Bajema

EXECUTIVE DIRECTOR Rachel Poarch

SOURCE BOOK EDITORIAL BOARD Rachel Bajema
Rachel Poarch
William M. Andrews
James Archer
Kimberly Battista
Alison Burke
Marie Dauenheimer
Jennifer Fairman
Peg Gerrity
Keith Kasnot
Maya Shoemaker
William Westwood

Medical Illustration & Animation 34
is produced and distributed by
**Serbin Creative, Inc. for the
Association of Medical Illustrators**

PRESIDENT / CREATIVE DIRECTOR Tamra Dempsey

MARKETING CONSULTANTS Ellie Altomare
Bryan Allen

PRODUCTION MANAGER Barbara Kuhn

BOOK DESIGN & PRODUCTION Terri Wright

DISTRIBUTION COORDINATOR Stacy Brostrom

ASSOCIATION OF MEDICAL ILLUSTRATORS For information on the profession of medical illustration or any member please contact:
Association of Medical Illustrators
Rachel Poarch, Executive Director
201 E. Main Street, Ste. 1405
Lexington, KY 40507
email: hq@ami.org
866-393-4264
www.ami.org

Special Thanks for Cover Image
Copyright © Melanie Connolly

Cover illustration: Depiction of the SARS-CoV-2 virus.

BACK COVER INSET IMAGES: (left to right)
Row 1 - Left, Nanbot Medical Scientific Communication; Right, Keri Leigh Biomedical Creations LLC
Row 2 - Left, Hofkin Studios
Middle, Biomedical Art; Right, Fairman Studios
Row 3 - Left, Fran Milner
Middle, Gerrity | Connolly - Chicago Medical Graphics
Right, subQstudio & Indiana Biosciences Research Institute/ Michael Pugia
Row 4 - Left, Bodell Medical Media; Middle, Lindsay MedArt

FACING PAGE: (left to right)
Scott Bodell, Bodell Medical Media;
Christoph Kuehne, 3-D.science;
Wenrong He;
Bill Blakesley, Neural Impulse Media

For information on advertising
or distribution please contact:
Serbin Creative, Inc.
110 N. Doheny Drive
Beverly Hills, CA 90211-1811
Tel: (805) 963-0439 or (800) 876-6425
hello@serbincreative.com

© 2021 Association of Medical Illustrators
Printed in Italy
ISBN: 978-1-883486-30-3
$50 USD

Medical Illustration & Animation 34 is published by the Association of Medical Illustrators. All rights reserved. No part of this book may be reproduced in any form or by any means, electronic or mechanical including photocopying, or stored in an information retrieval system without the prior written permission of the Association of Medical Illustrators.

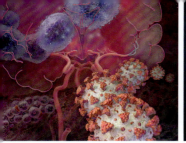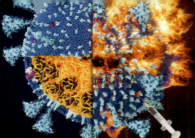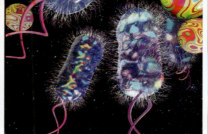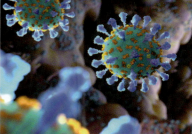

An Historic Year for Medical Illustration

This year marked one of the most urgent challenges in modern medical illustration:
How to illustrate a pandemic.

Members of the Association of Medical Illustrators took collaboration to new heights this year. We shared research, newly released 3D structural models of the envelope proteins, and everything else we discovered about the virus's structure and mechanics in an open-source repository.

The images we created have helped define our collective experience and visual memories of this historic time.

When the first images coming out of the National Institutes of Health went viral the demand for new content went sky-high. Medical illustrators raced to collaborate with researchers to help uncover the structure of the novel coronavirus COVID-19, then worked and re-worked artistic concepts as new science emerged. We helped explain the virus's mechanism of infection and how to prevent its spread. We partnered with innovators to patent new types of PPE, explained how the vaccine candidates work, and re-conceptualized health care spaces to better accommodate highly infectious patient populations. This was a massive community undertaking to educate the public and attempt to save lives.

Medical illustrators were proud to be part of this fight, hoping our contributions helped to stem the tide of mounting infection rates and public anxiety. You'll see many examples of this work in the following pages, and more using searchable keywords on the portfolio website **www.medillsb.com**.

During this overwhelming time, we have also looked inward, as a continued focus on global diversity and inclusion influenced conversations around representation in medical art. As we grow, our profession continues to draw vibrant, diverse visual communicators to our ranks, and it has been a joy to draw attention to the inclusive representation in the work we make, allowing us to continue learning, honing our artistic sense of editorship, making better, more useful art, and celebrating our diverse global membership and client base.

We look forward to working with you in telling next year's stories. We look to 2021 with hope, celebrating science that has provided protection and served humankind, and continuing to ask hard questions, search for new ideas, and explaining the best of these through art.

Rachel Bajema, MS, CMI

Editor

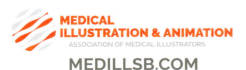

MEDILLSB.COM

🐦 medillustrates
📷 medicalillustration
📘 medillsb
📷 medical.animation
💼 medical-illustration-&-animation

contents

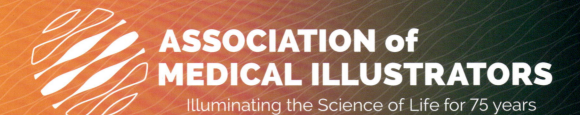

ASSOCIATION of MEDICAL ILLUSTRATORS

Illuminating the Science of Life for 75 years

©2020 Audra Geras   ©2020 Emily Cheng   ©2019 Hang Lin

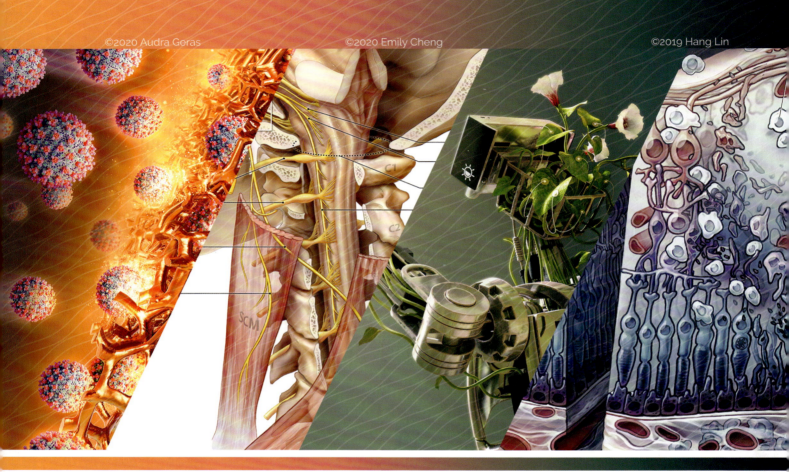

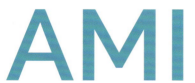 inspires a diverse community of innovators in biomedical visualization to apply their creativity, scientific expertise, and communication skills toward making a difference in the world, advancing scientific discovery, and improving healthcare literacy.

See more award-winning work by our members at ami.org

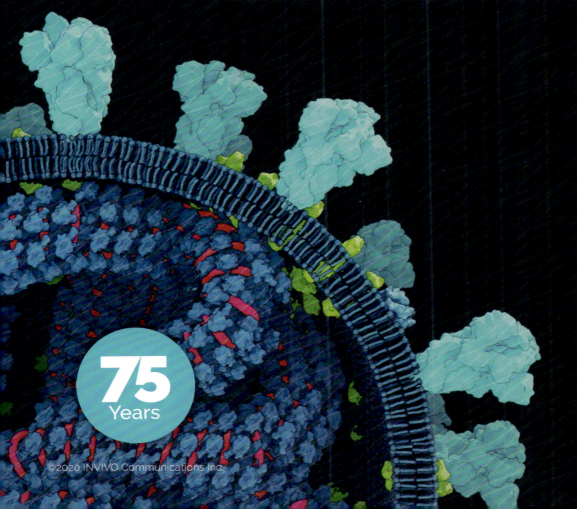

Science Matters.
Data Matter.
Facts Matter.
Diversity Matters.
Visuals Matter.

Certification Matters.

Hire board-certified medical illustrators & animators.

75 Years

C·M·I
BOARD
CERTIFIED
MEDICAL
ILLUSTRATOR

©2020 INVIVO Communications Inc.

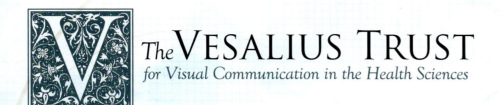

The VESALIUS TRUST
for Visual Communication in the Health Sciences

Recognizing excellence.
Preserving the legacy.
Building a future together.

SUPPORTING EXCELLENCE IN HEALTH SCIENCE VISUAL COMMUNICATIONS

The Vesalius Trust, founded in 1988, fosters the study, research, and practice in visual communication of health information at all levels. From childhood through the practice of medicine and cutting-edge research, learning from quality imagery is increasingly important in today's high-energy digital world.

Join us! However you can give, we thank you for your support.

SUPPORT OUR MISSION

Visit VesaliusTrust.org

vt@vesaliustrust.org
+1 (904) 878-7801

View artist portfolios online at

MEDILLSB.COM

View artist portfolios online at

MEDILLSB.COM

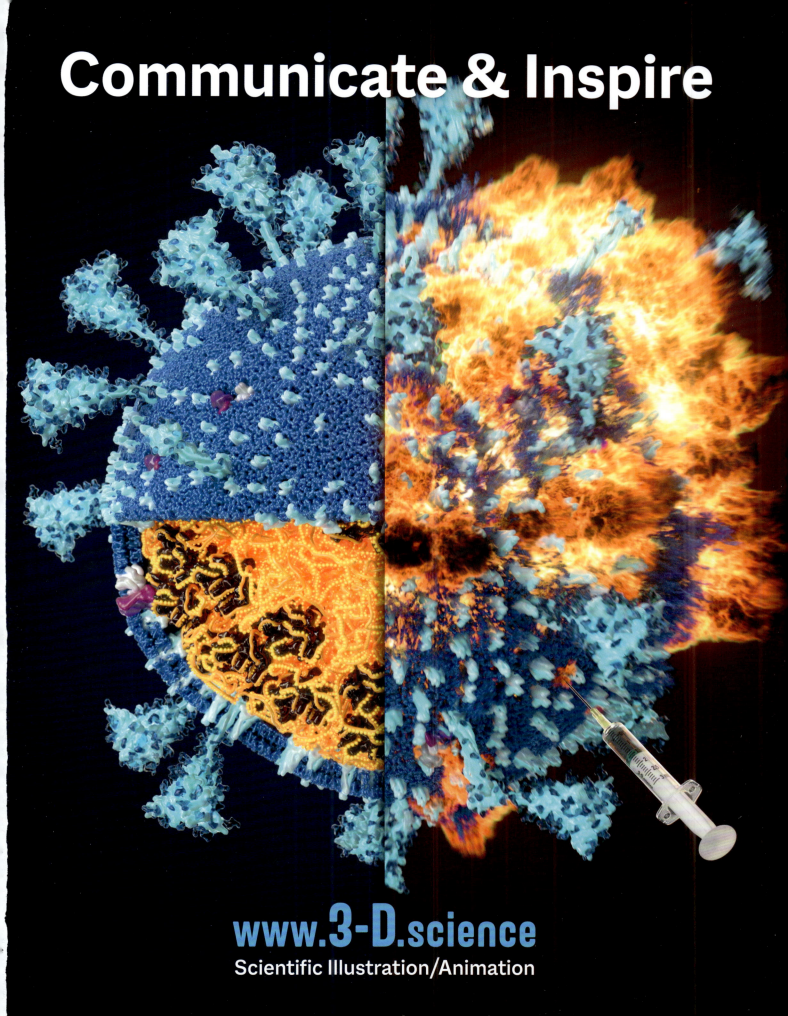

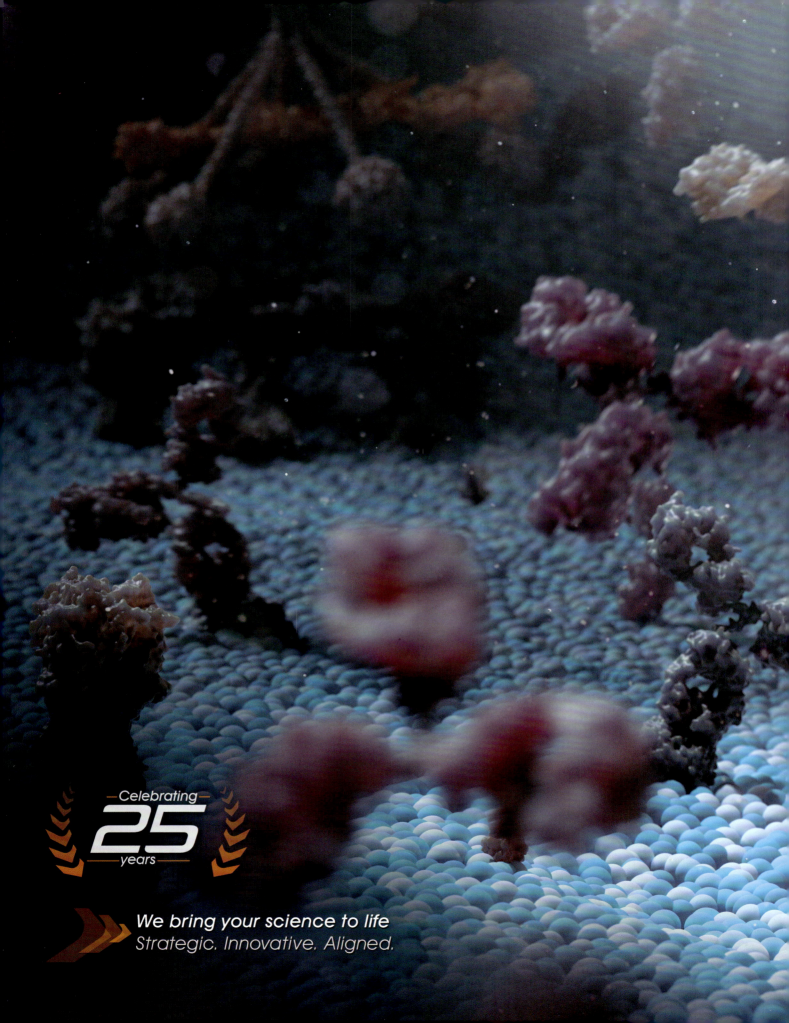

Celebrating 25 years

We bring your science to life
Strategic. Innovative. Aligned.

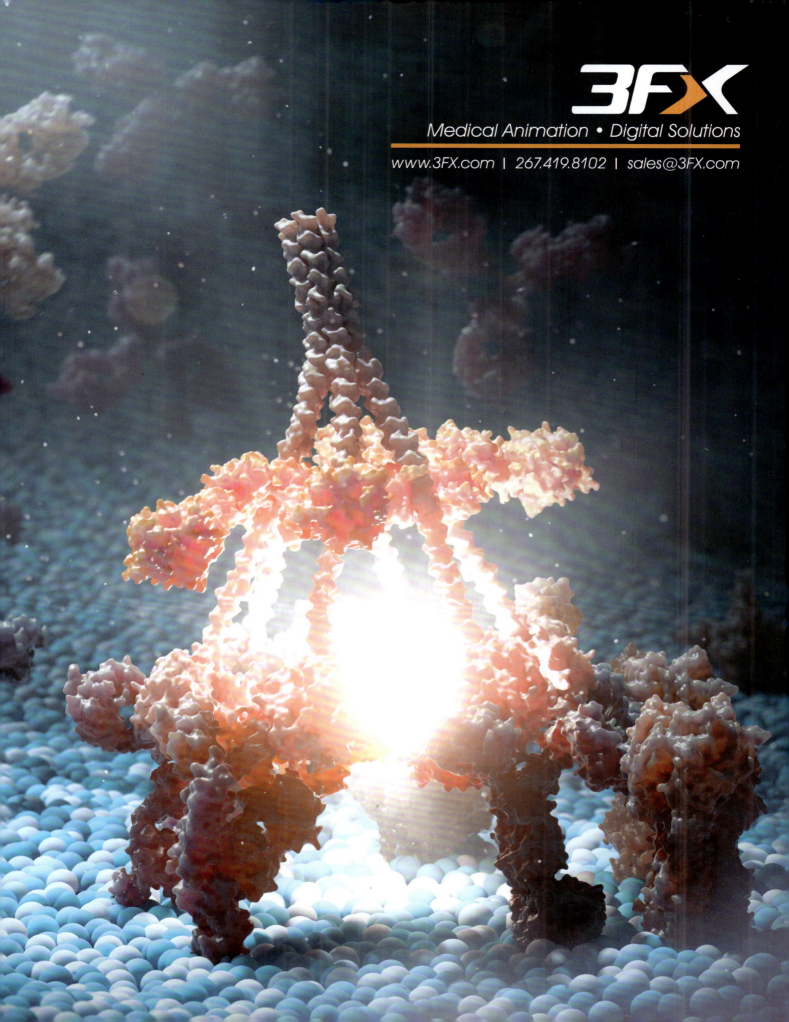

3FX

Medical Animation • Digital Solutions

www.3FX.com | 267.419.8102 | sales@3FX.com

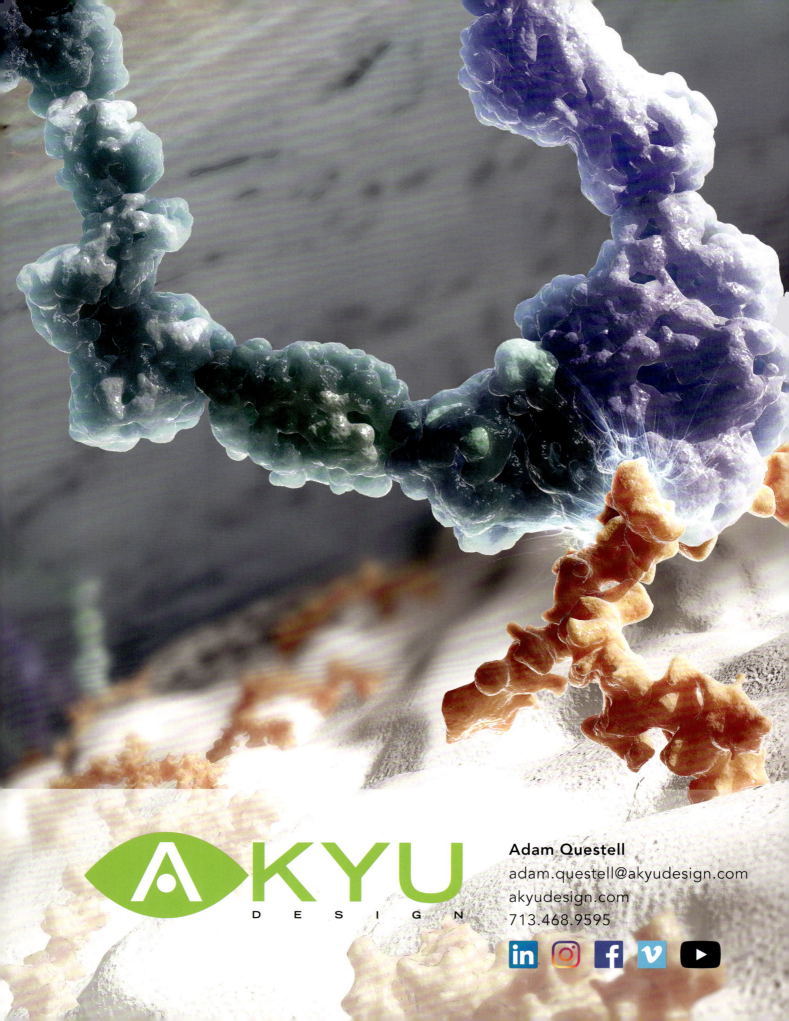

AKYU
DESIGN

Adam Questell
adam.questell@akyudesign.com
akyudesign.com
713.468.9595

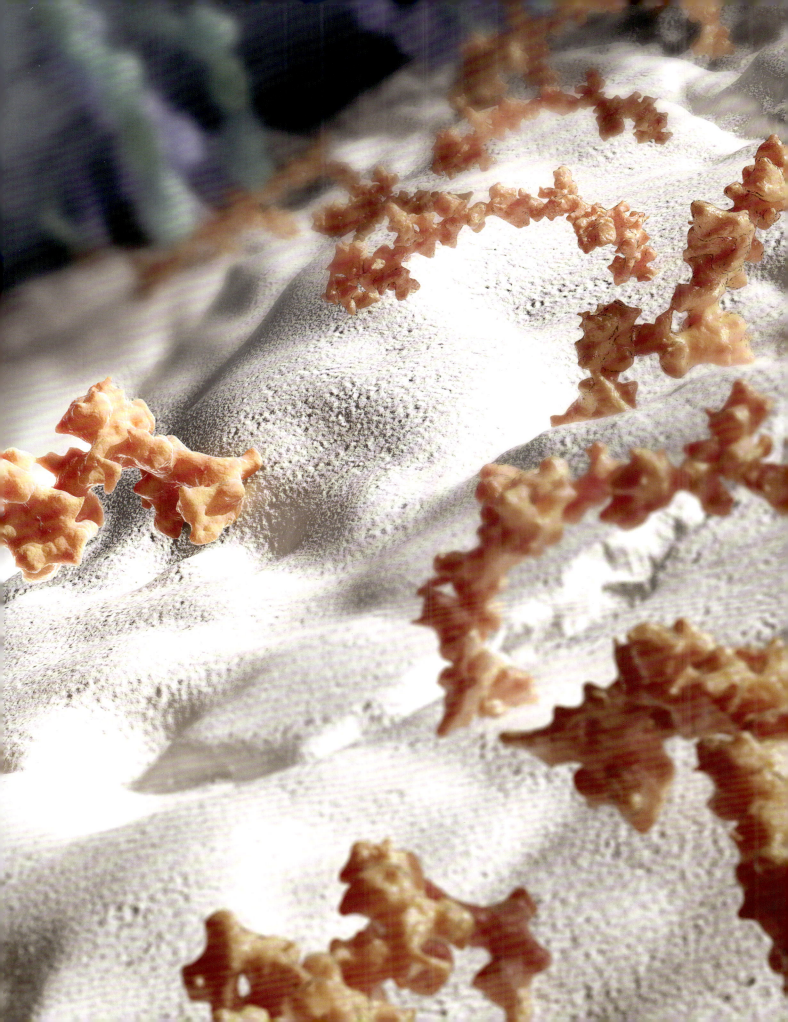

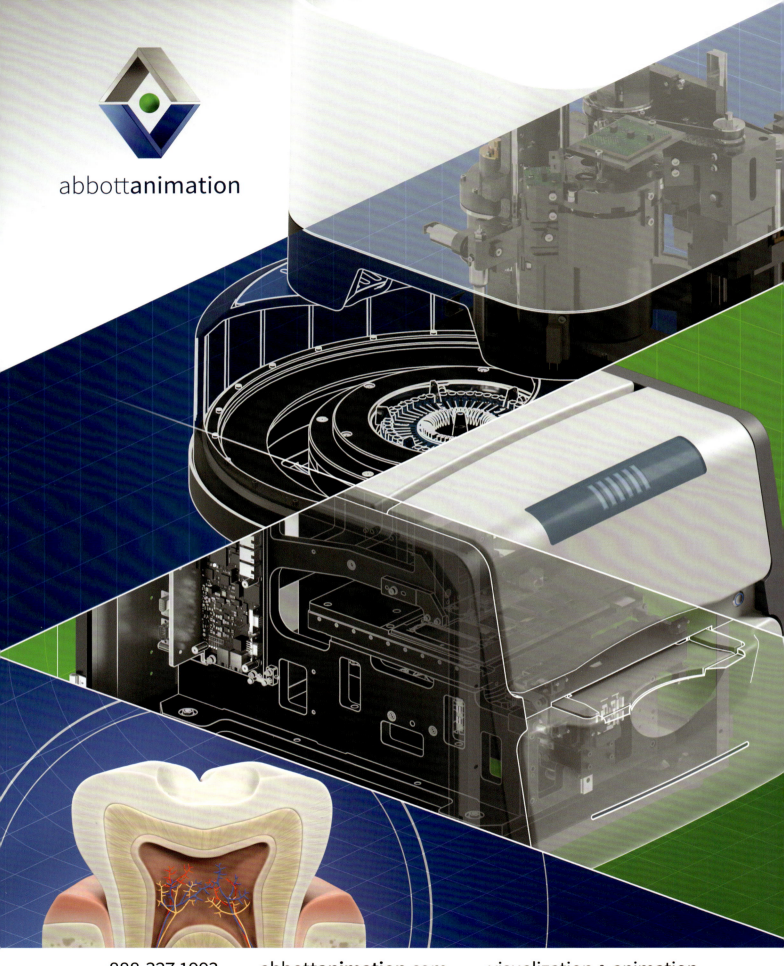

888-327-1993   •   abbott**animation**.com   •   visualization & animation

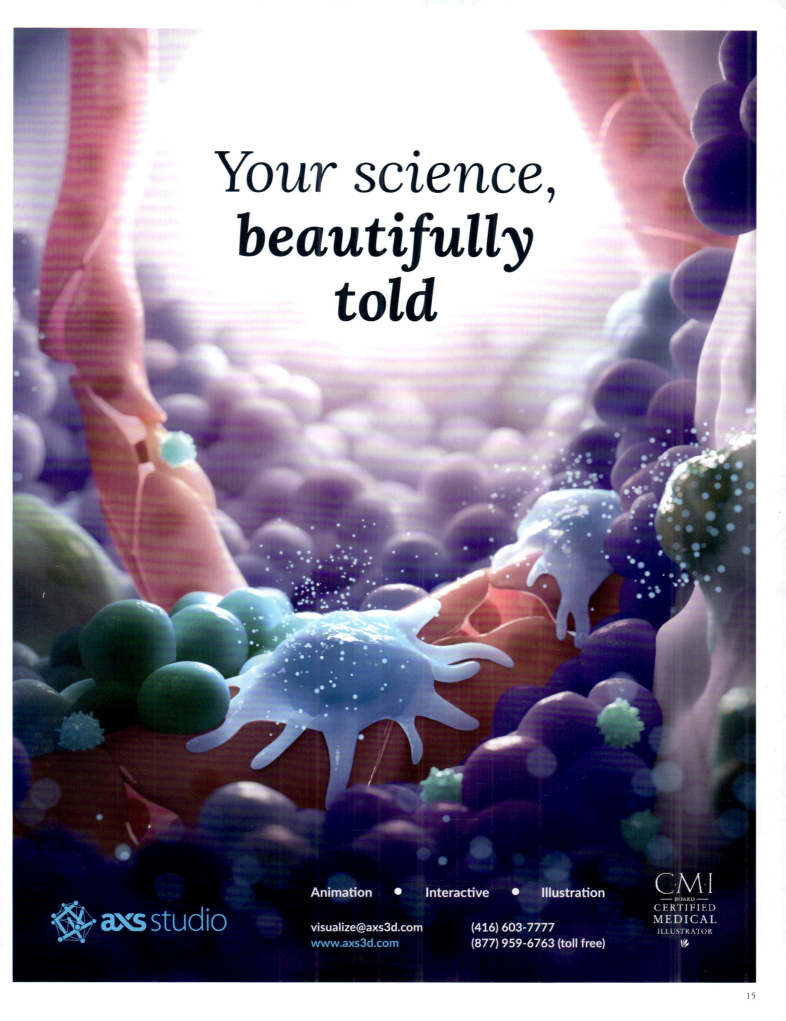

Your science, beautifully told

Animation • Interactive • Illustration

axs studio

visualize@axs3d.com
www.axs3d.com

(416) 603-7777
(877) 959-6763 (toll free)

CMI
BOARD
CERTIFIED
MEDICAL
ILLUSTRATOR

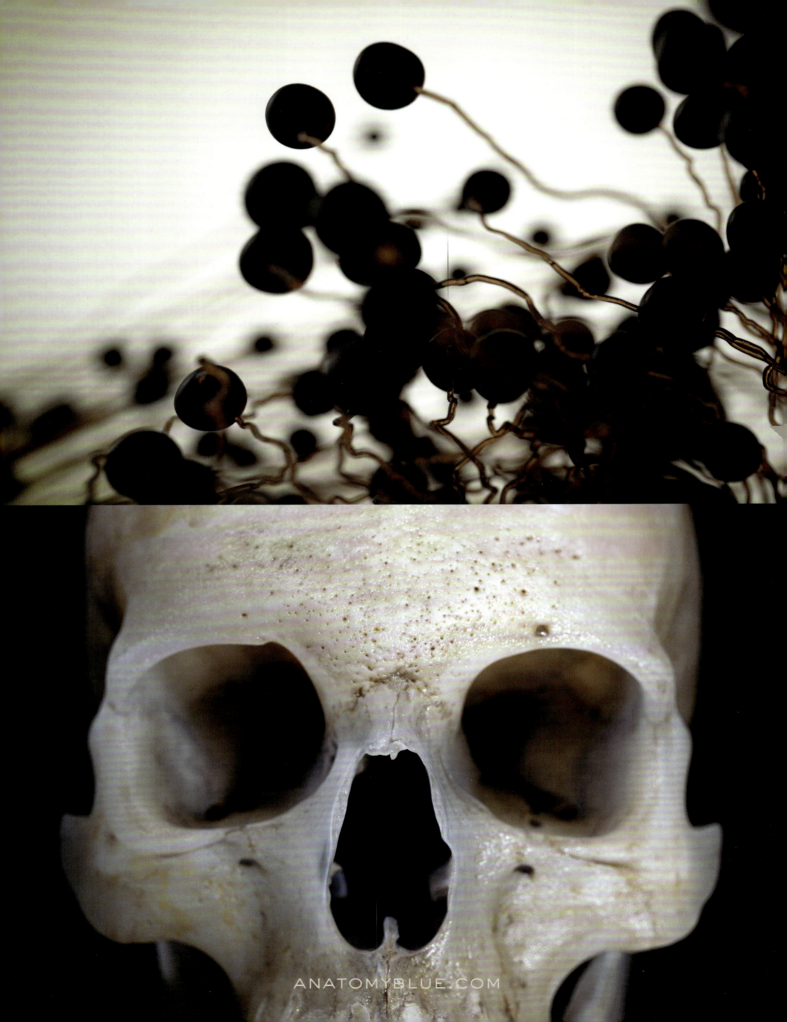

ANATOMYBLUE.COM

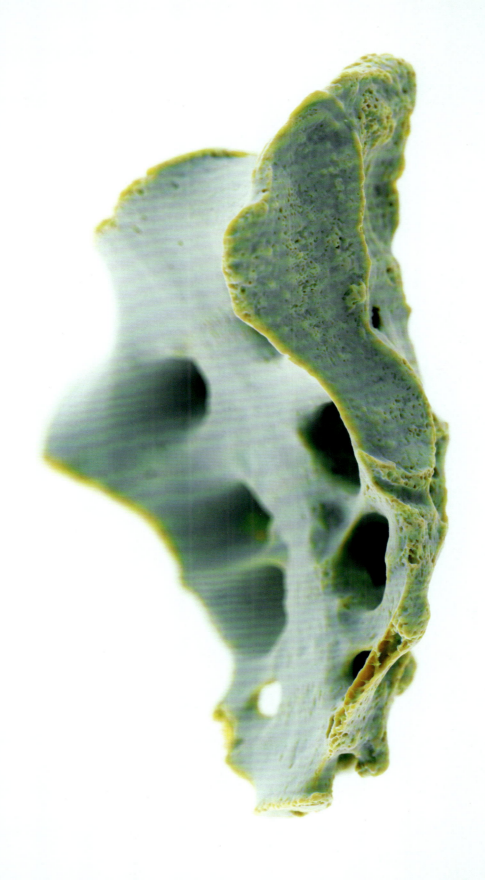

ANATOMYBLUE

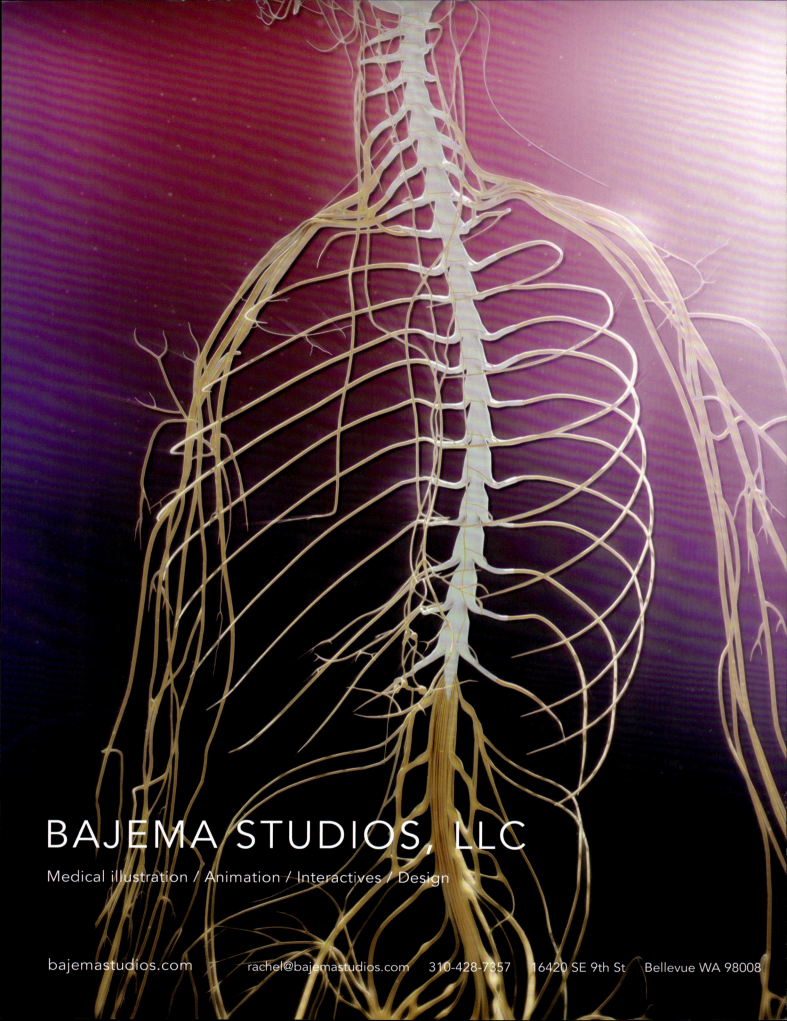

BAJEMA STUDIOS, LLC

Medical illustration / Animation / Interactives / Design

bajemastudios.com   rachel@bajemastudios.com   310-428-7357   16420 SE 9th St   Bellevue WA 98008

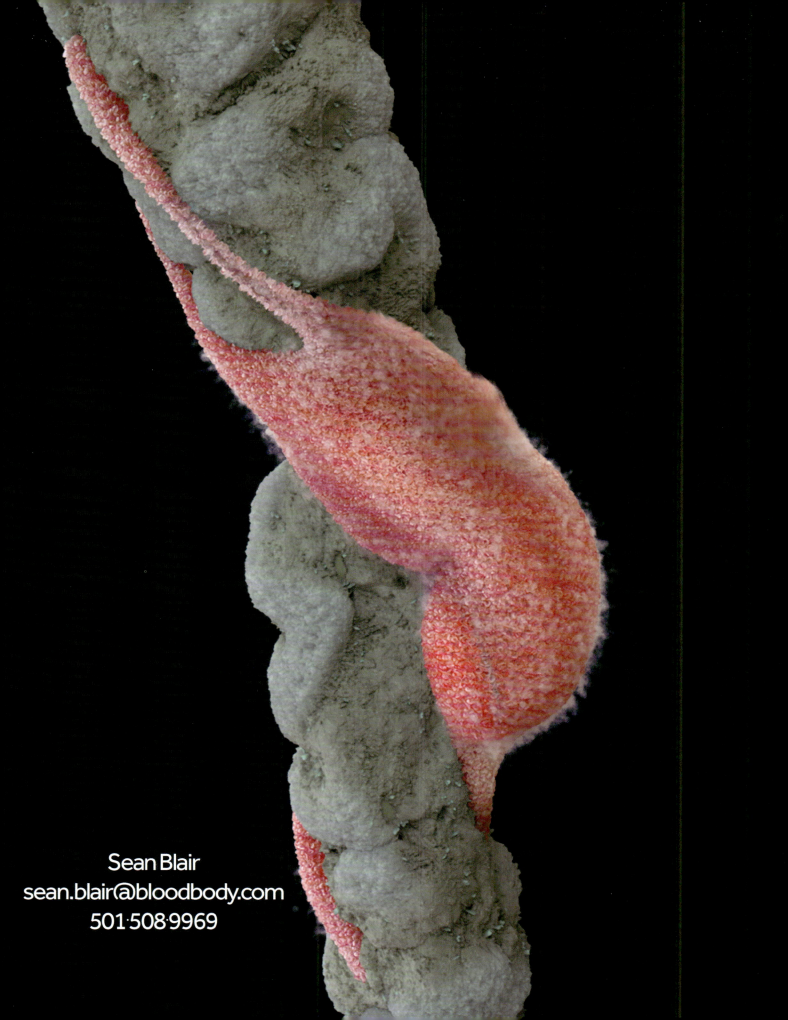

Sean Blair
sean.blair@bloodbody.com
501·508·9969

OUR CHARACTER DRIVEN ANIMATIONS INCREASE ENGAGEMENT AND UNDERSTANDING, HELPING TO COMMUNICATE MEDICAL CONCEPTS IN THE MOST EFFECTIVE WAY POSSIBLE.

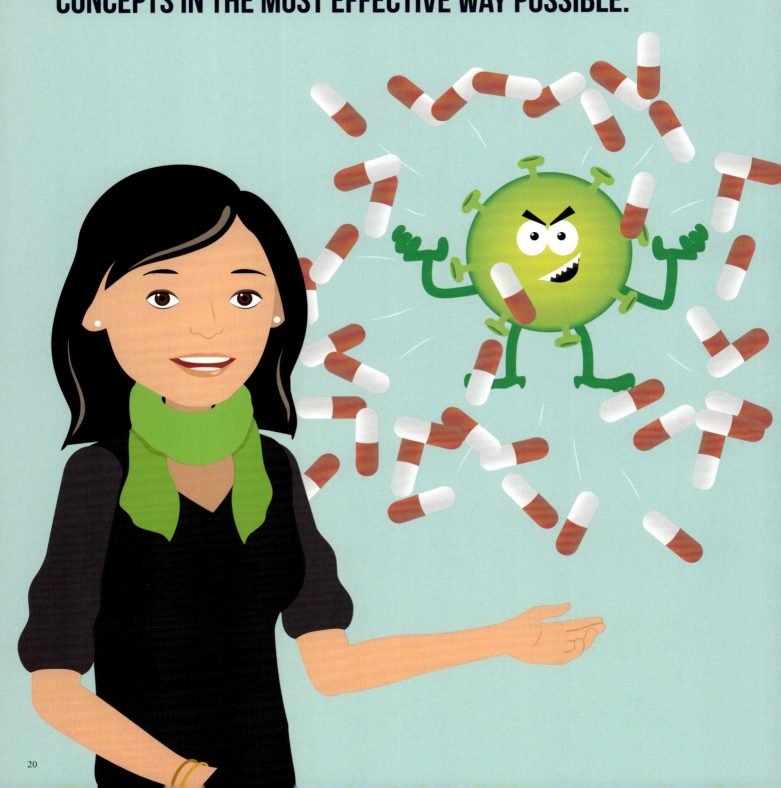

BELUGA
ANIMATION

WE COMBINE THE

SCIENCE OF COMMUNICATION

WITH THE

ART OF ANIMATION

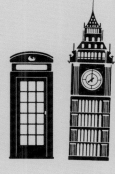

BASED IN LONDON, ENGLAND

GET IN TOUCH: HELLO@BELUGAANIMATION.COM

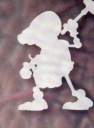

BREAKIRON®
Animation&Design

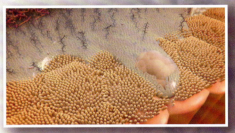

00:00:48

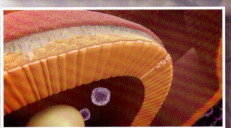

00:00:55

00:01:08

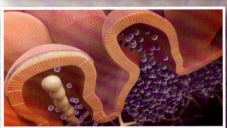

00:01:43

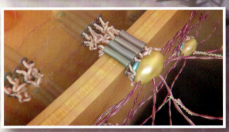

00:02:03

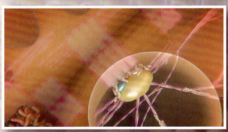

00:02:40

Life
Animated
Visualized
Illustrated

On target, on time and on budget.

www.breakiron.com

919.523.8414

COMMERCIAL • **MEDICAL** • FILM • MOTION GRAPHICS
▲

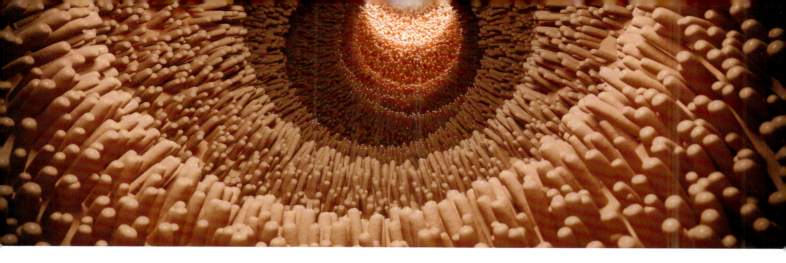

PAUL BROWN

MEDICAL/SCIENTIFIC VISUALIZATION SERVICES

MOA/MOD • DEVICES • SIMULATIONS • AR • VR

hello@paulbrownv.com

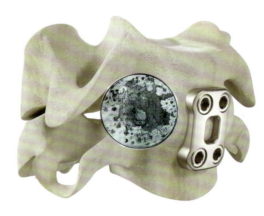
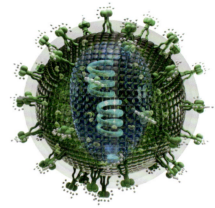
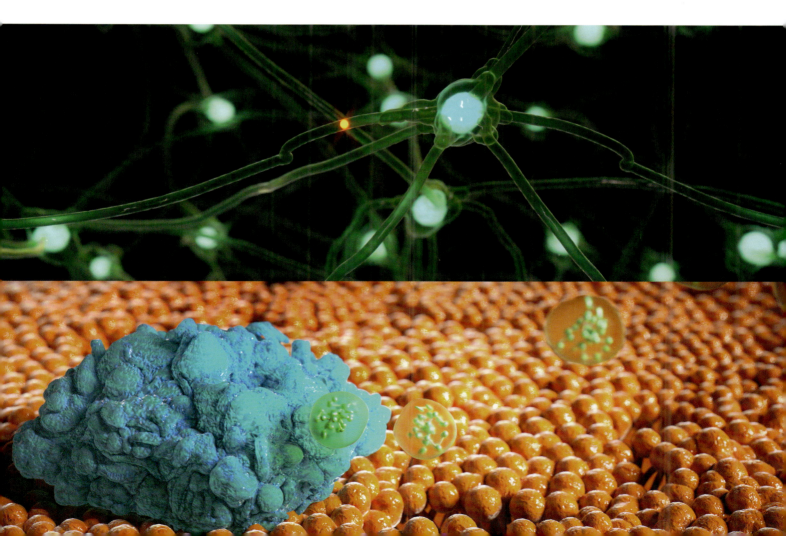

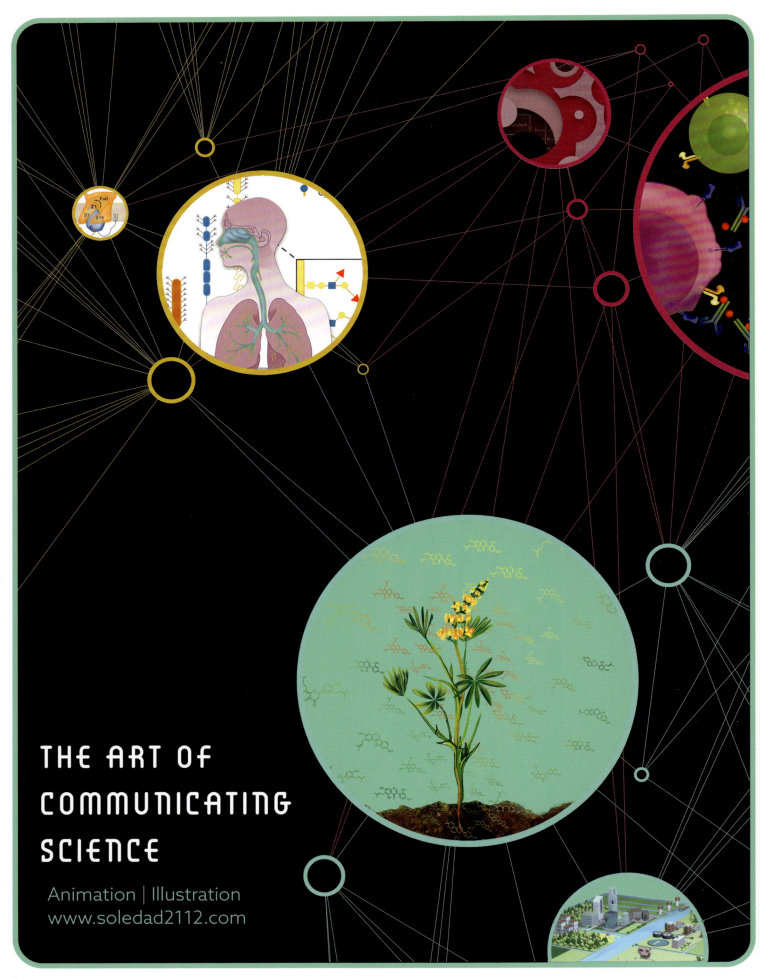

THE ART OF COMMUNICATING SCIENCE

Animation | Illustration
www.soledad2112.com

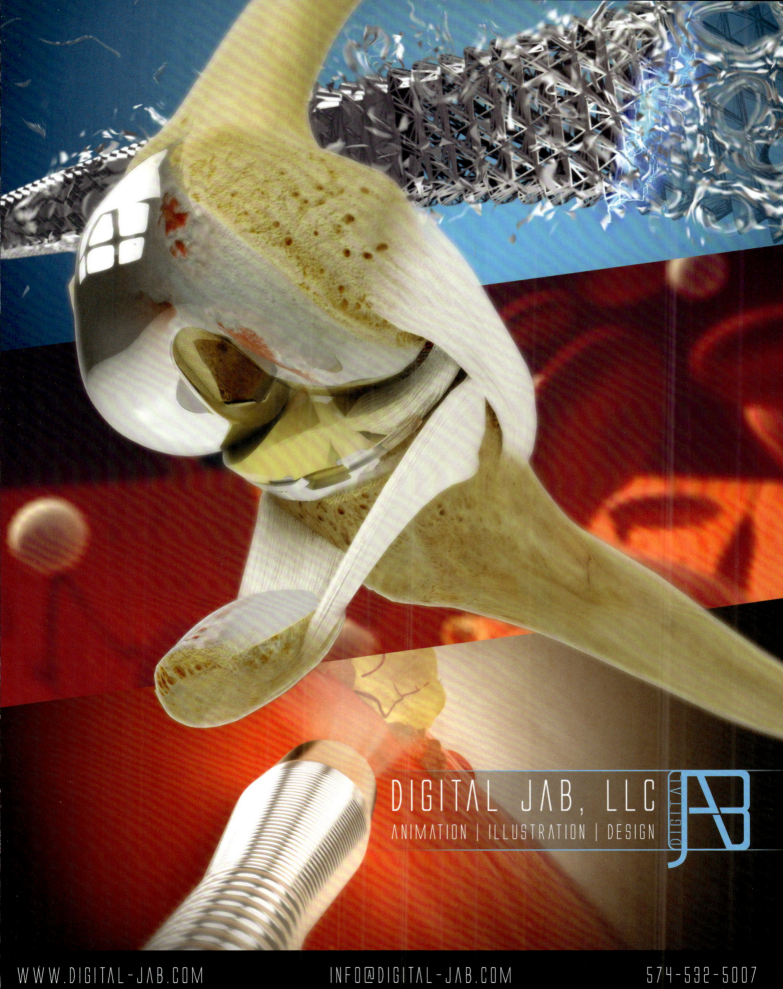

DIGITAL JAB, LLC
ANIMATION | ILLUSTRATION | DESIGN

WWW.DIGITAL-JAB.COM INFO@DIGITAL-JAB.COM 574-532-5007

ENCEPHALO CREATIVE

Biomedical Creativity

Creating impactful visual media to bring complex scientific & medical content to life.

INTERACTIVE MEDIA   MEDICAL LEGAL   DESIGN

EncephaloCS@gmail.com

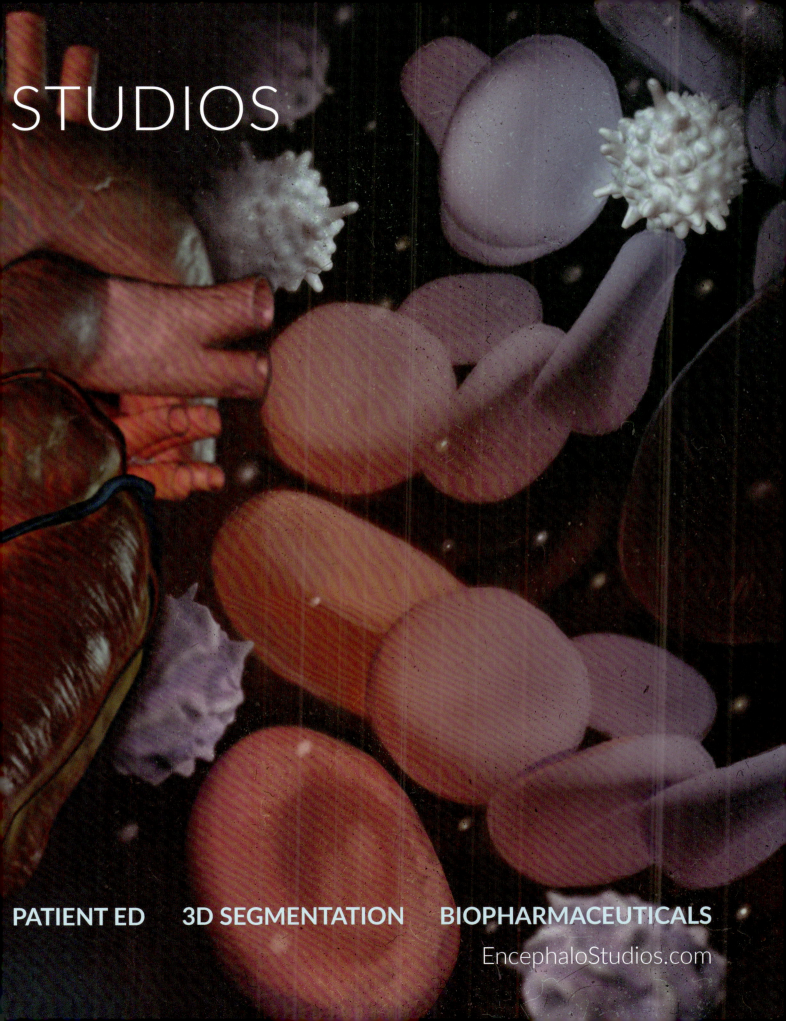

STUDIOS

PATIENT ED   3D SEGMENTATION   BIOPHARMACEUTICALS

EncephaloStudios.com

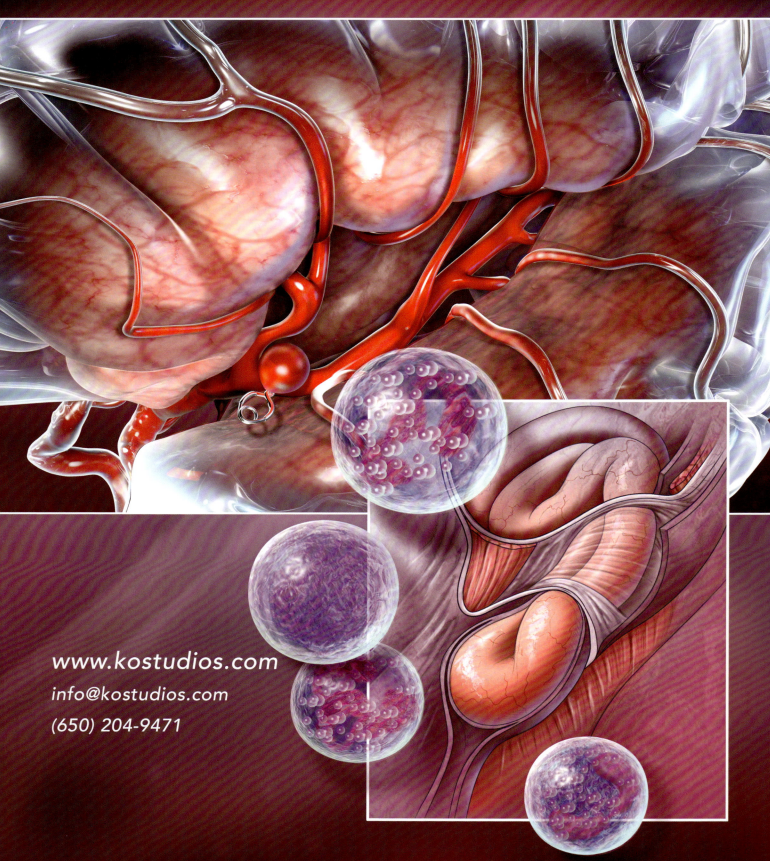

KO STUDIOS

Medical Animation and Illustration

www.kostudios.com

info@kostudios.com

(650) 204-9471

All images ©KO Studios 2021. All rights reserved.

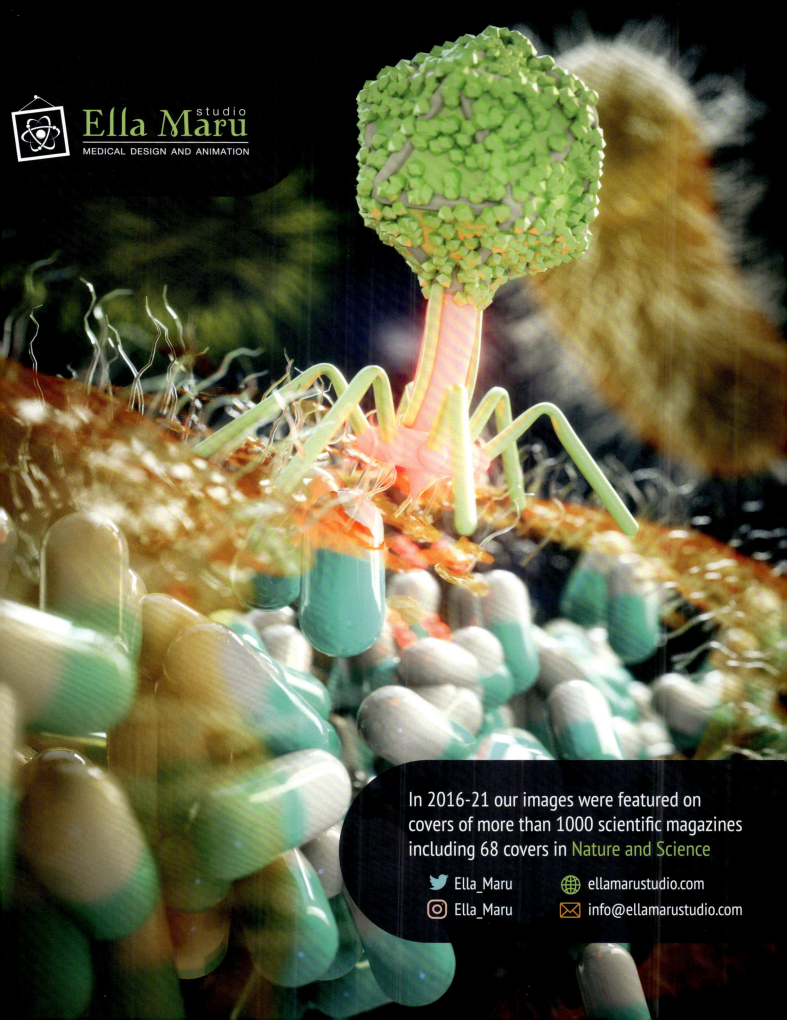

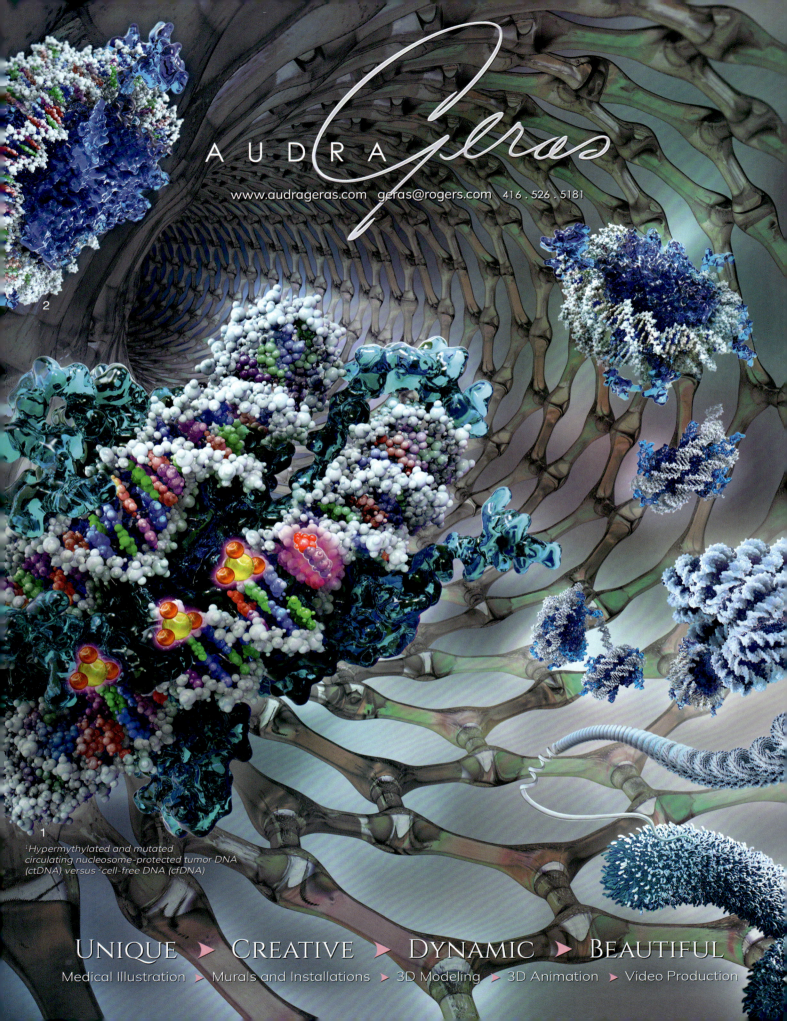

AUDRA Geras

www.audrageras.com   geras@rogers.com   416 . 526 . 5181

¹Hypermythylated and mutated
circulating nucleosome-protected tumor DNA
(ctDNA) versus ²cell-free DNA (cfDNA)

UNIQUE ▶ CREATIVE ▶ DYNAMIC ▶ BEAUTIFUL
Medical Illustration ▶ Murals and Installations ▶ 3D Modeling ▶ 3D Animation ▶ Video Production

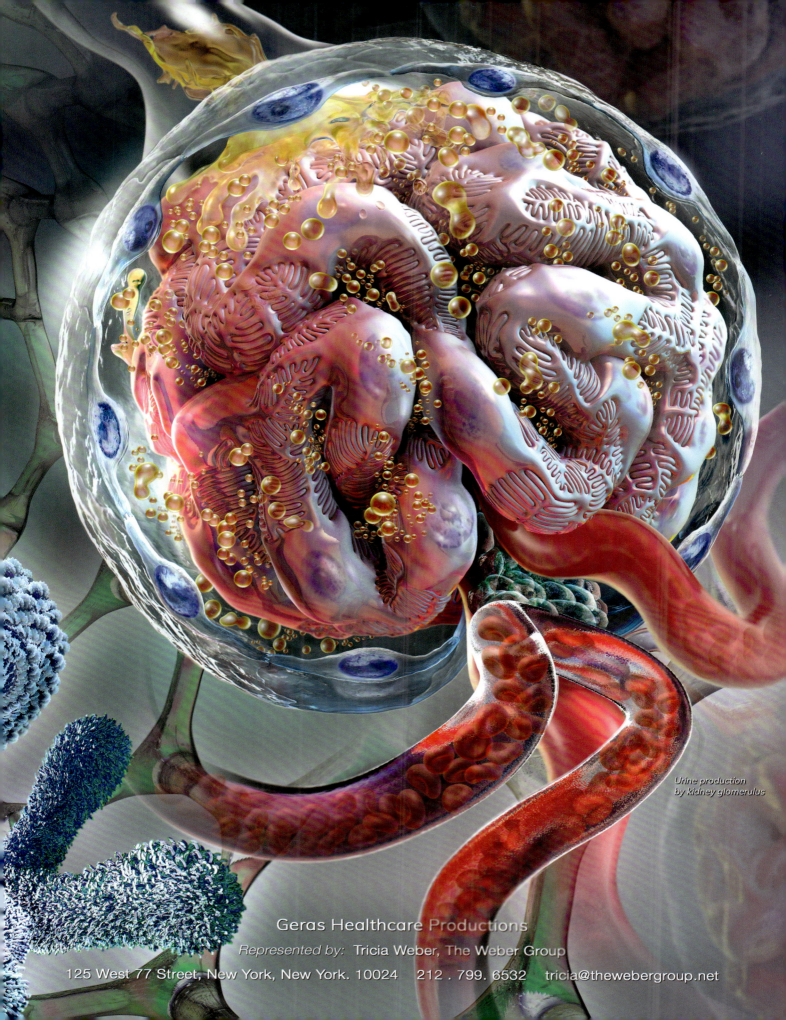

*Urine production
by kidney glomerulus*

Geras Healthcare Productions

Represented by: Tricia Weber, The Weber Group

125 West 77 Street, New York, New York. 10024   212 . 799 . 6532   tricia@thewebergroup.net

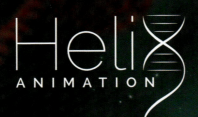

mRNA

RNA polymerase

DNA

DNA Transcription

Devoted to supporting healthcare
research teams & awareness initiatives
in their noble cause to create
a better tomorrow

www.helixanimation.com

SPELLBINDING I IMMENSELY ACCURATE I COST-EFFECTIVE

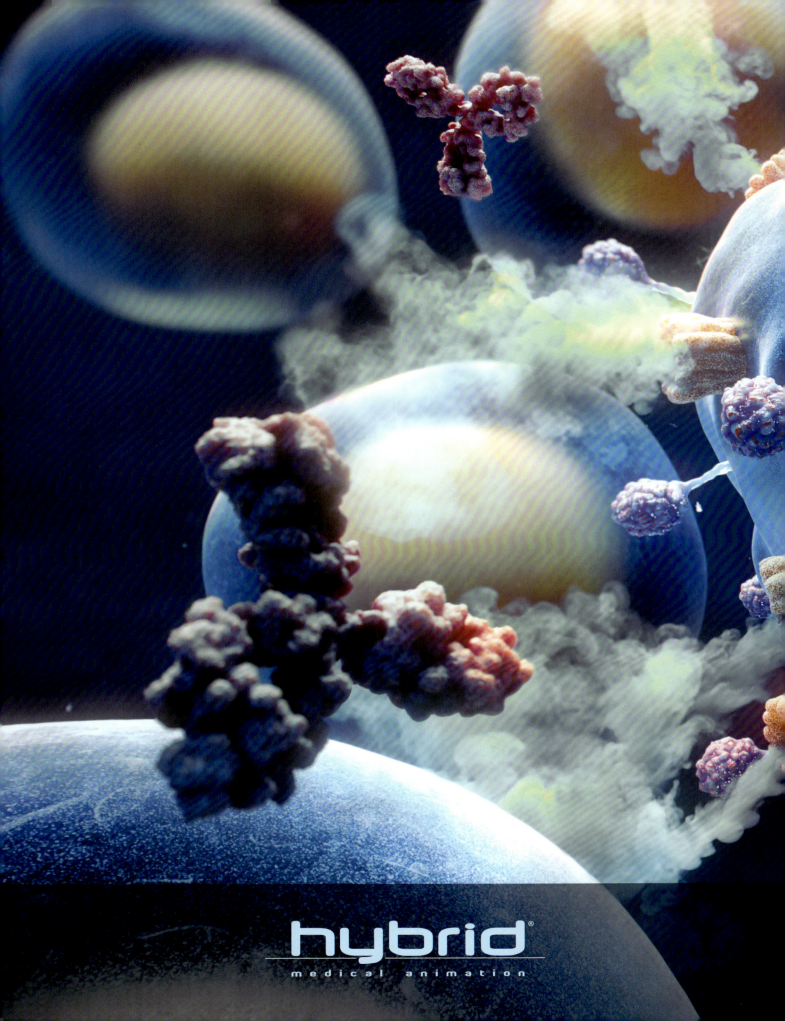

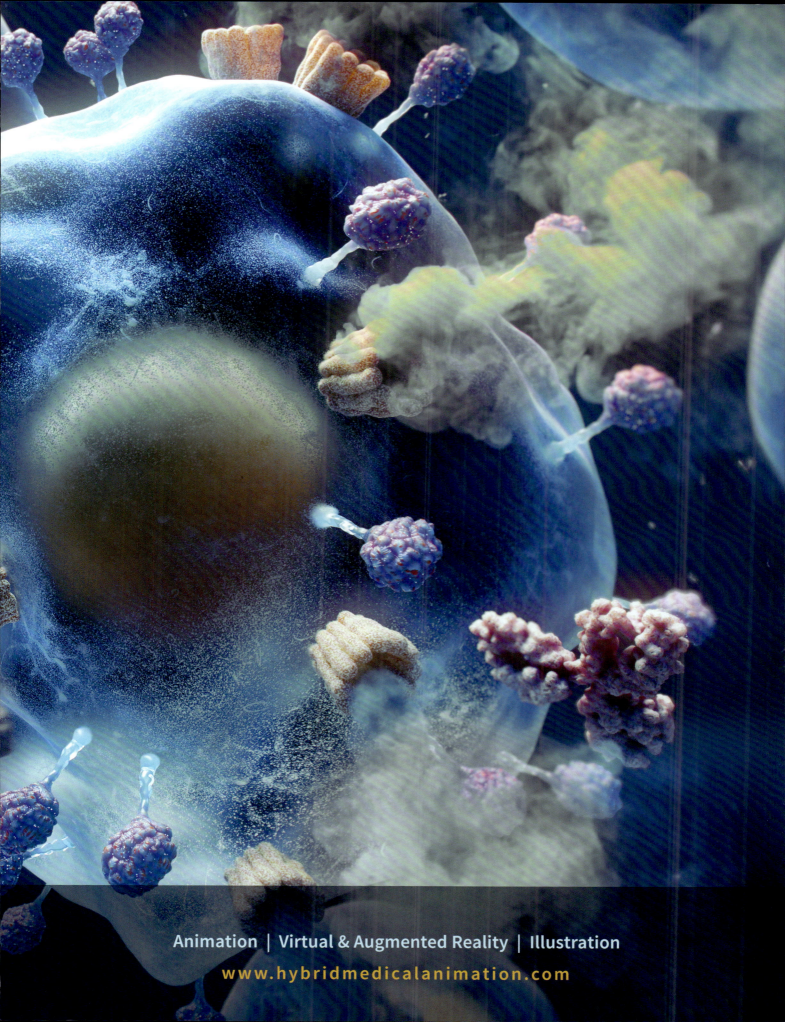

Animation | Virtual & Augmented Reality | Illustration
www.hybridmedicalanimation.com

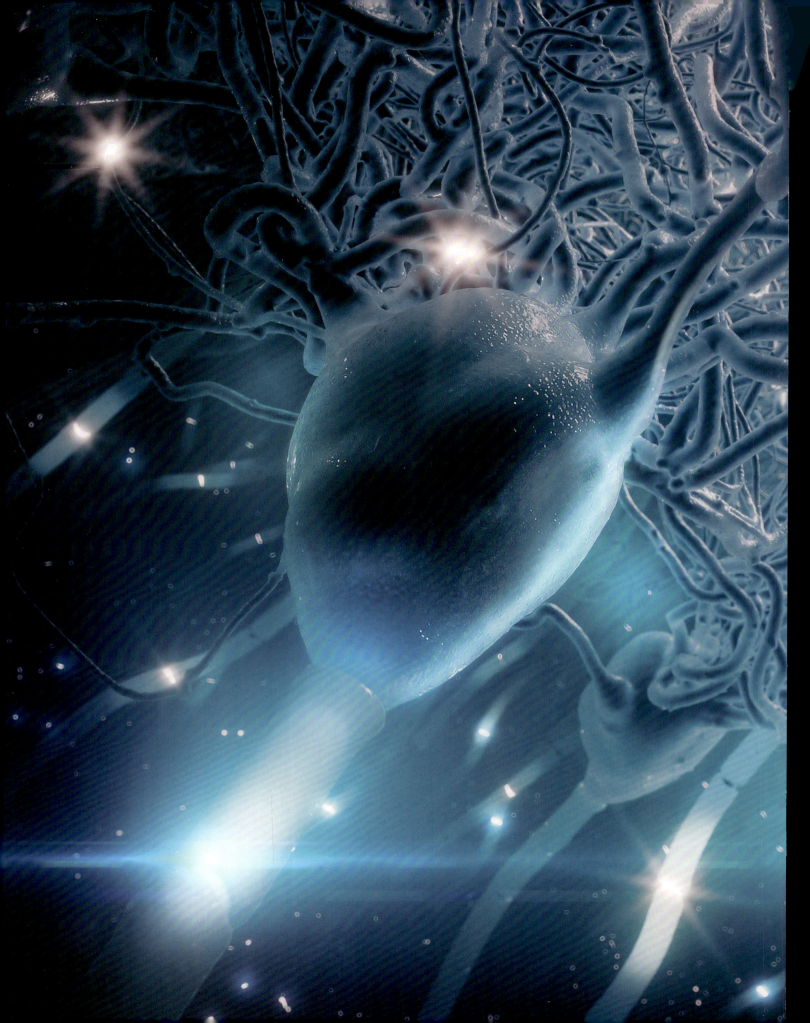

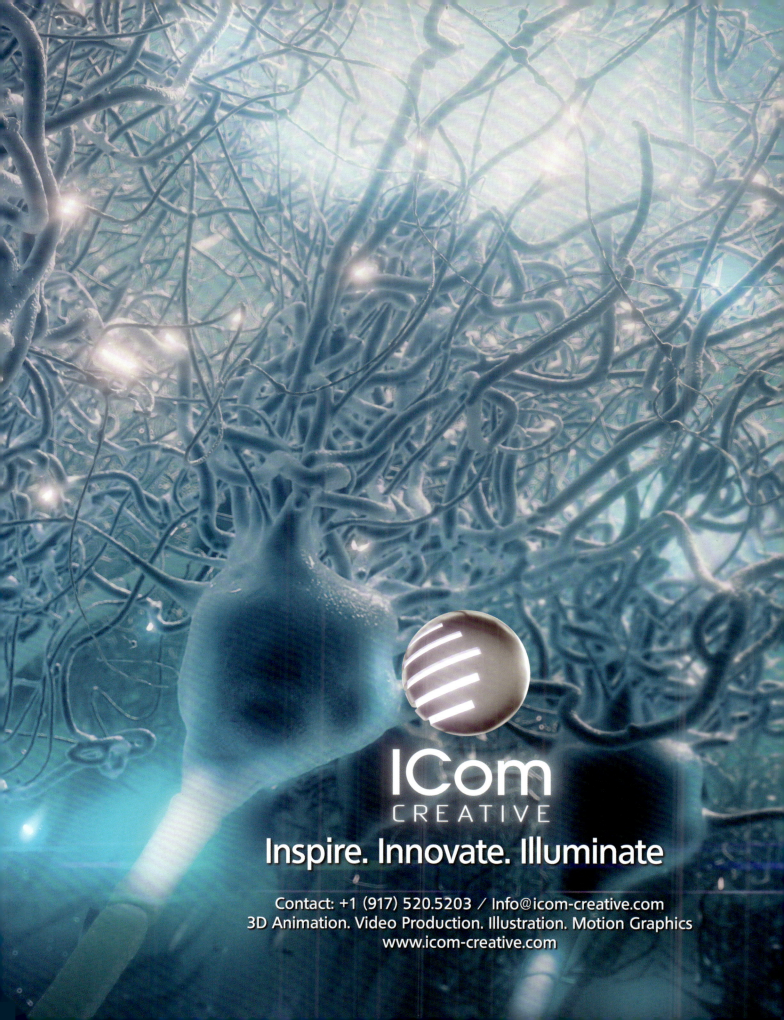

ICom
CREATIVE
Inspire. Innovate. Illuminate

Contact: +1 (917) 520.5203 / Info@icom-creative.com
3D Animation. Video Production. Illustration. Motion Graphics
www.icom-creative.com

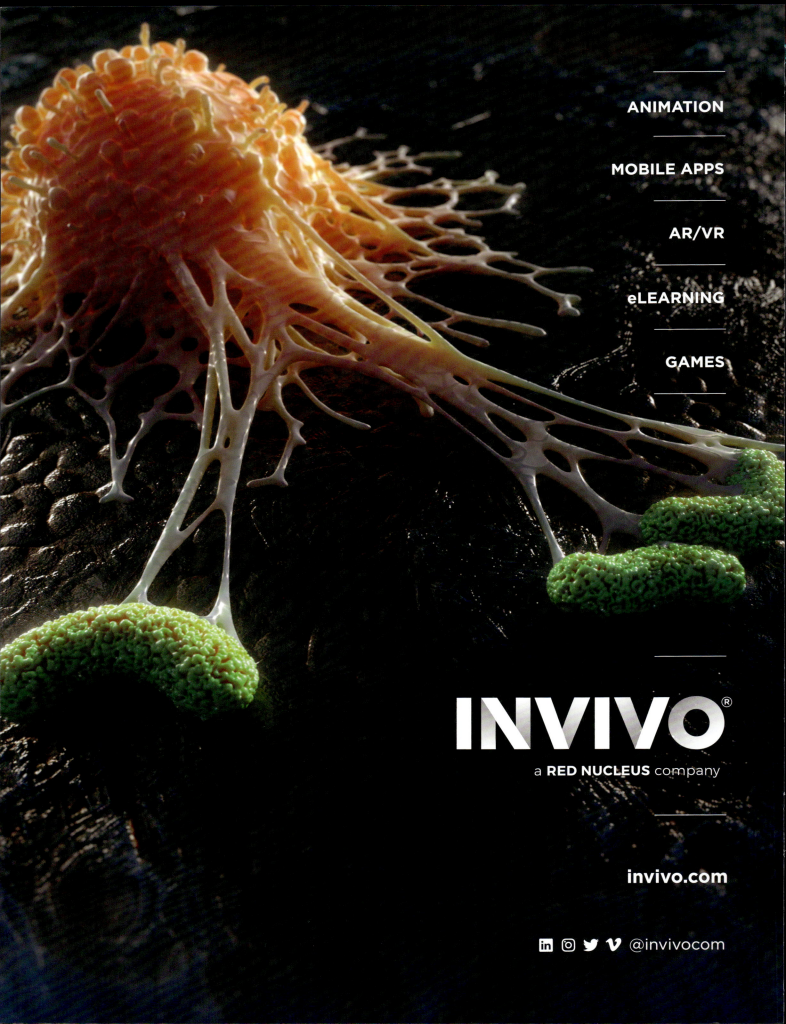

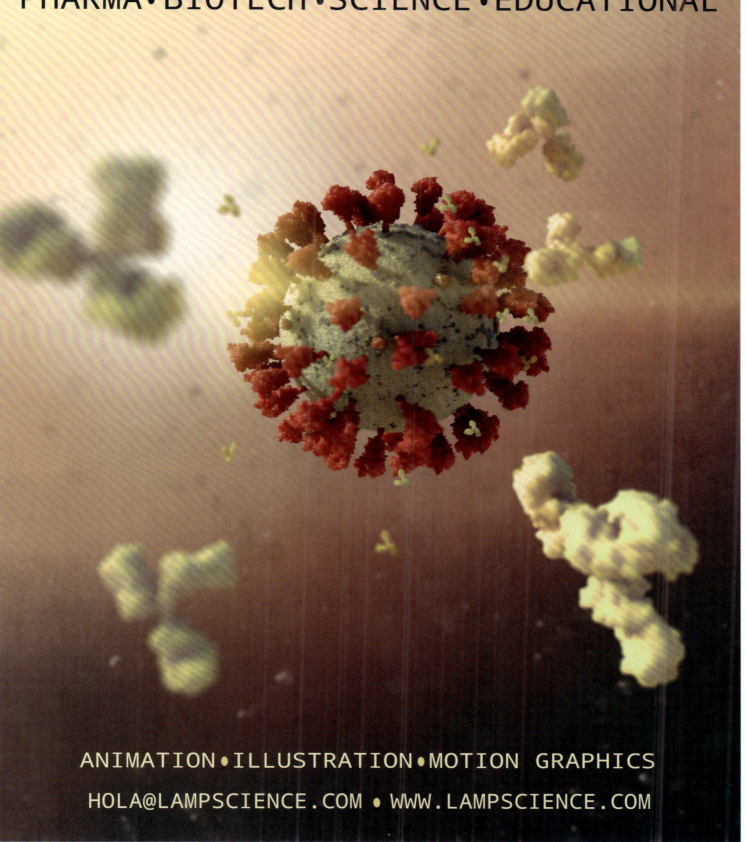

PHARMA•BIOTECH•SCIENCE•EDUCATIONAL

ANIMATION•ILLUSTRATION•MOTION GRAPHICS

HOLA@LAMPSCIENCE.COM • WWW.LAMPSCIENCE.COM

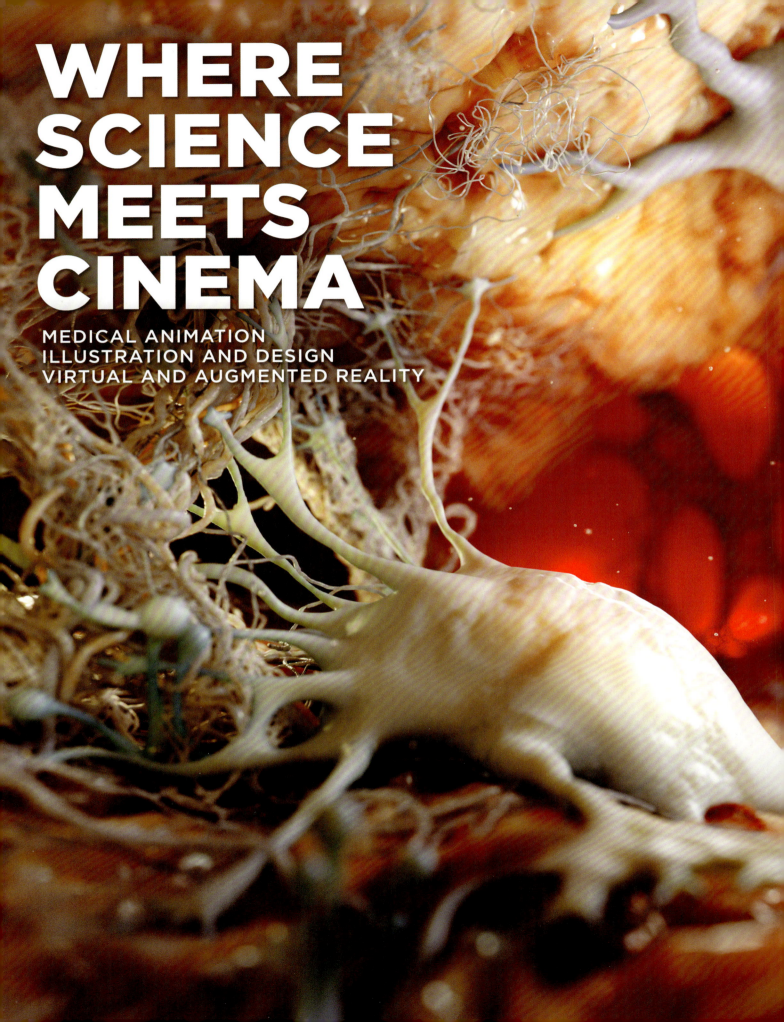

WHERE
SCIENCE
MEETS
CINEMA

MEDICAL ANIMATION
ILLUSTRATION AND DESIGN
VIRTUAL AND AUGMENTED REALITY

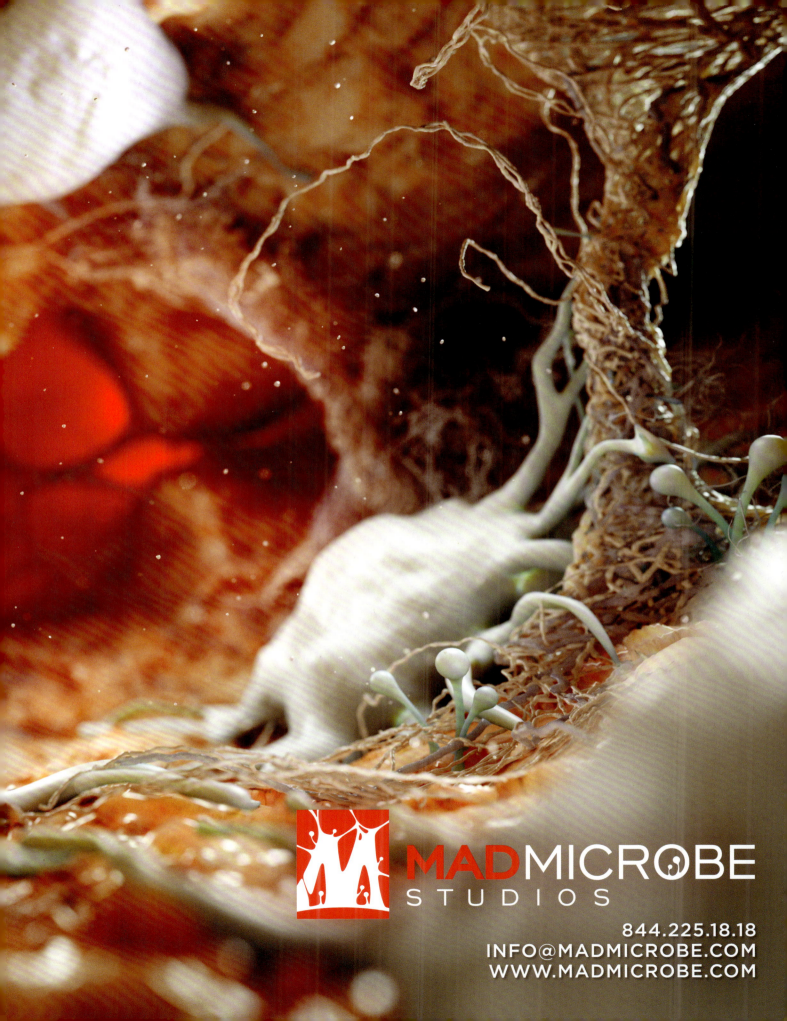

MADMICROBE
STUDIOS

844.225.18.18
INFO@MADMICROBE.COM
WWW.MADMICROBE.COM

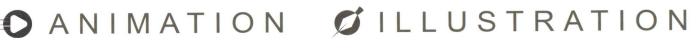
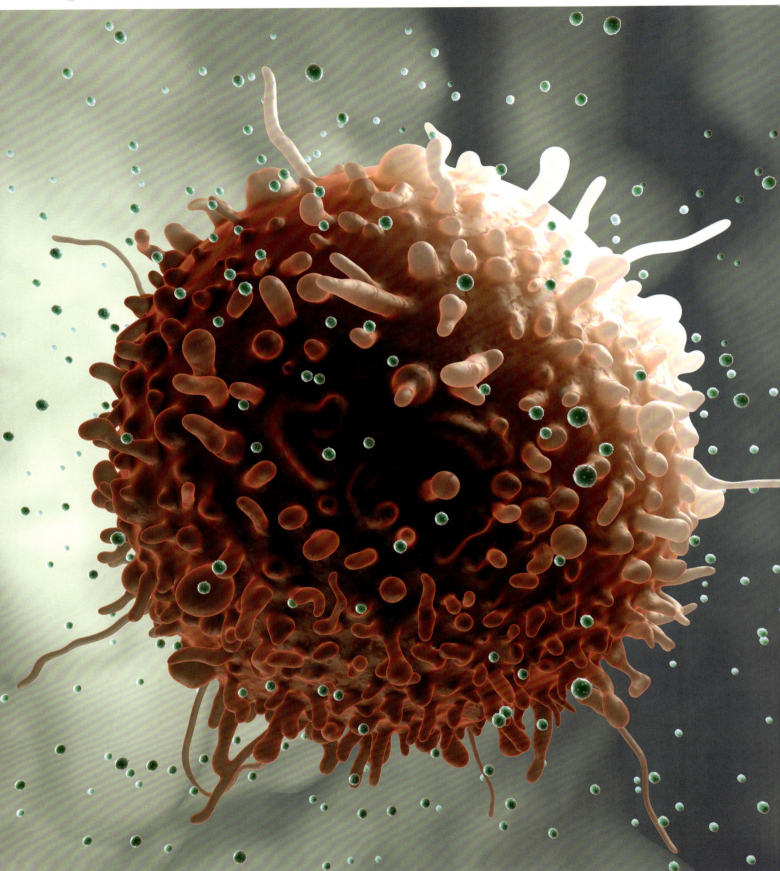

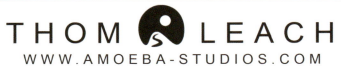
THOM   LEACH
WWW.AMOEBA-STUDIOS.COM

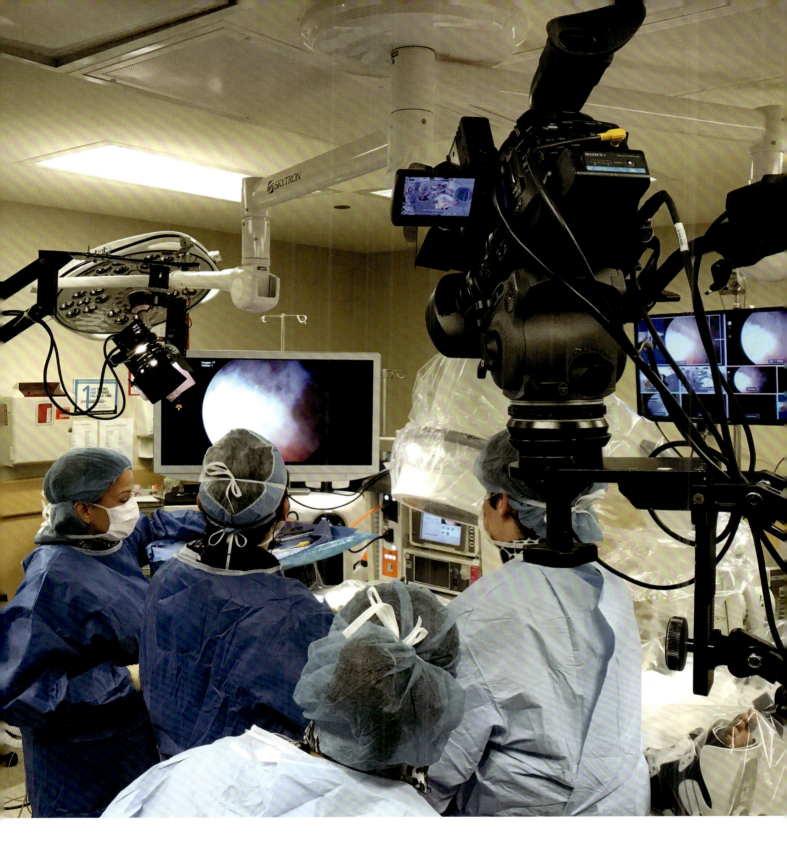

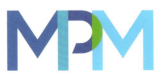
mpmfirst.com
info@mpmfirst.com

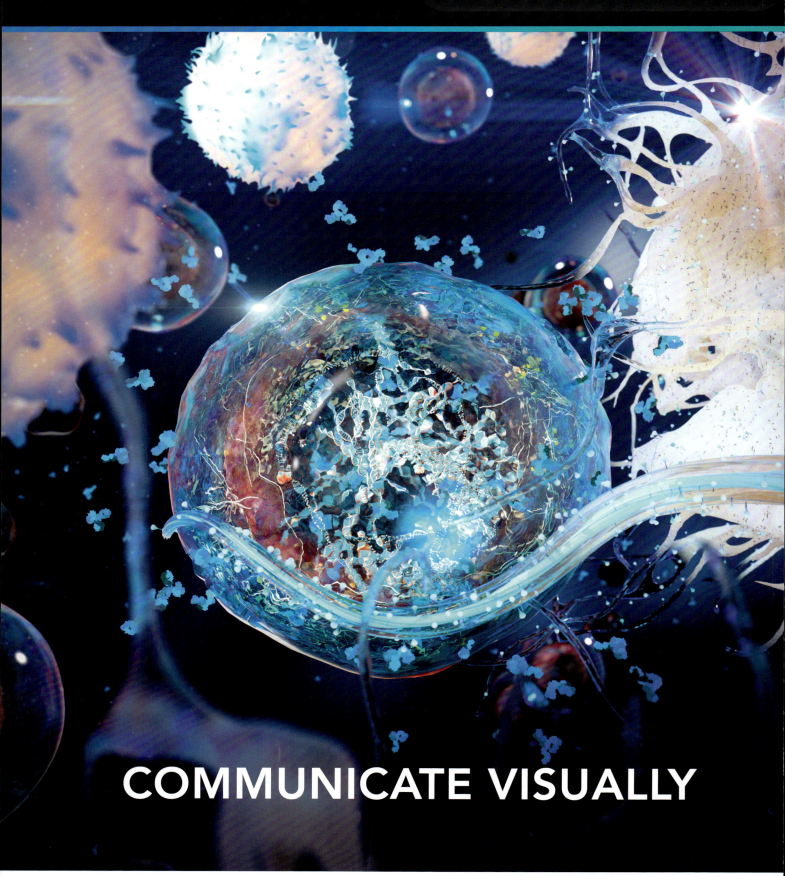

NANOBOT MEDICAL COMMUNICATION

3D Animation • 3D Illustration • Web • VR/AR • Interactive

Our website:
www.nanobotmedical.com

+1 858 207 87 81
y.svidinenko@nanobotmedical.com

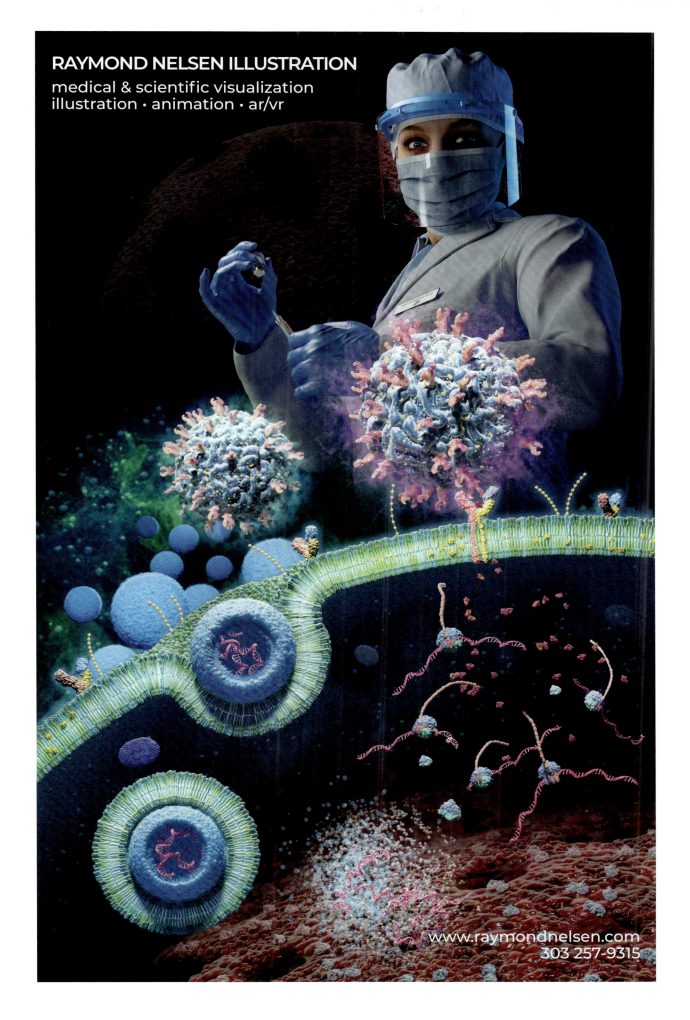

RAYMOND NELSEN ILLUSTRATION

medical & scientific visualization
illustration · animation · ar/vr

www.raymondnelsen.com
303 257-9315

45

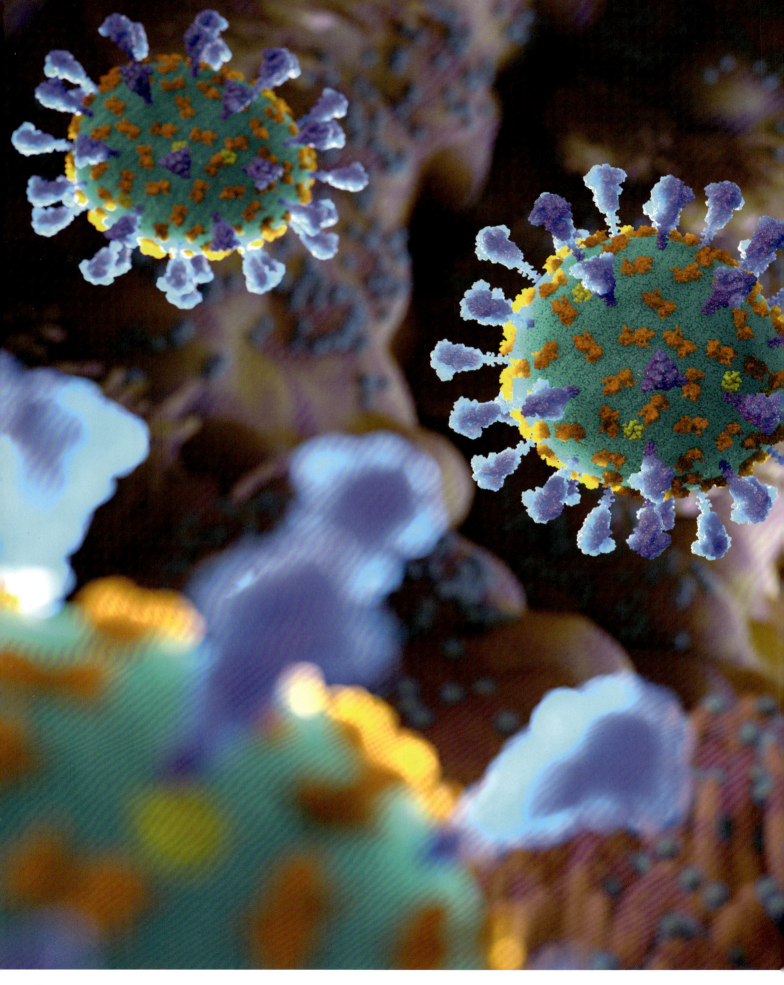

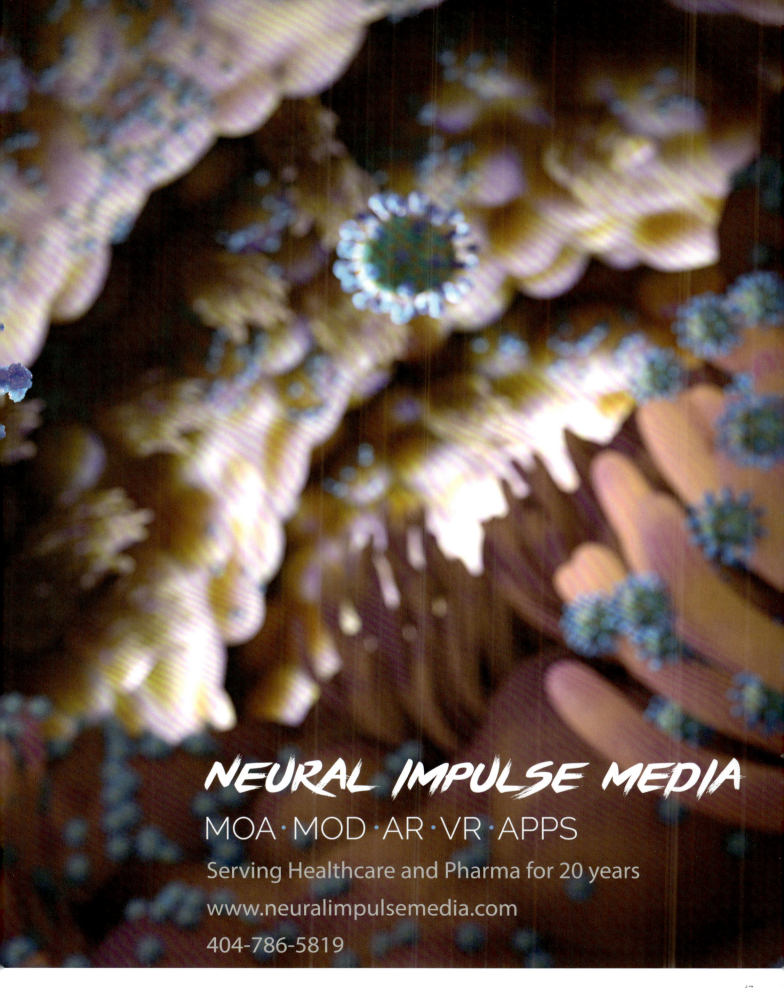

NEURAL IMPULSE MEDIA

MOA · MOD · AR · VR · APPS

Serving Healthcare and Pharma for 20 years

www.neuralimpulsemedia.com

404-786-5819

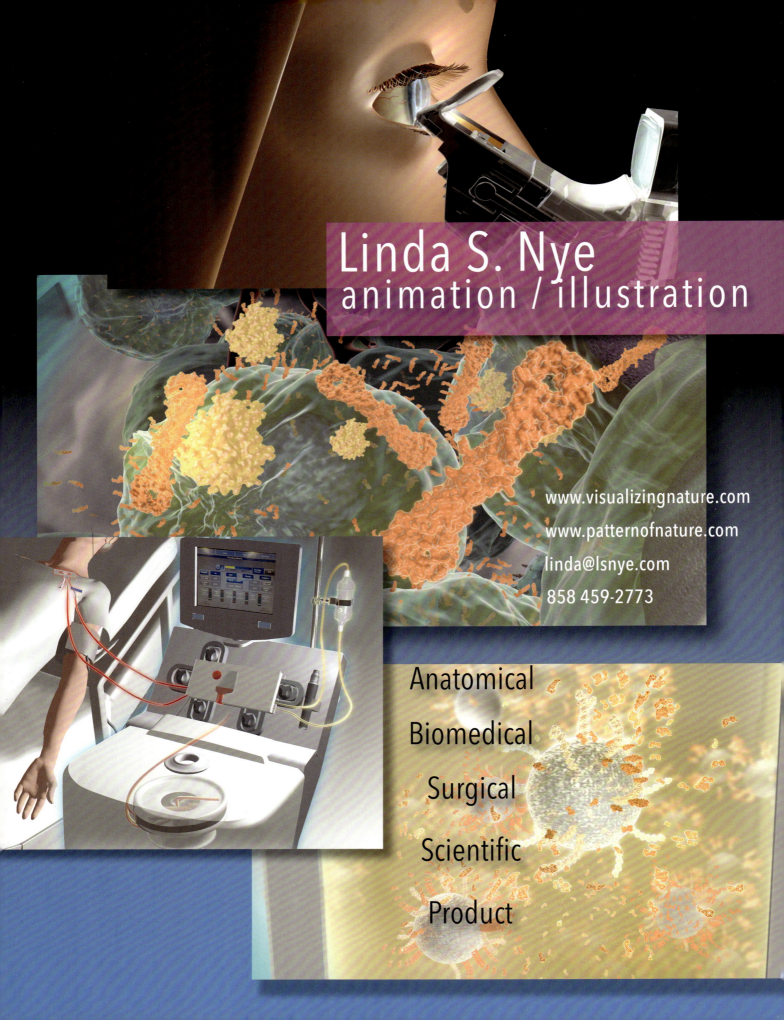

Linda S. Nye
animation / illustration

www.visualizingnature.com
www.patternofnature.com
linda@lsnye.com
858 459-2773

Anatomical

Biomedical

Surgical

Scientific

Product

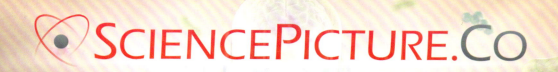

**COMPLEX SCIENCE
BEAUTIFULLY CAPTURED**

ANIMATION . ILLUSTRATION . VR . STOCK

An award winning 3D medical animation studio renowned for creating
cinematic 3D visualizations in the fields of medicine, science and technology.

info@sciencepicturecompany.com | www.sciencepicture.co

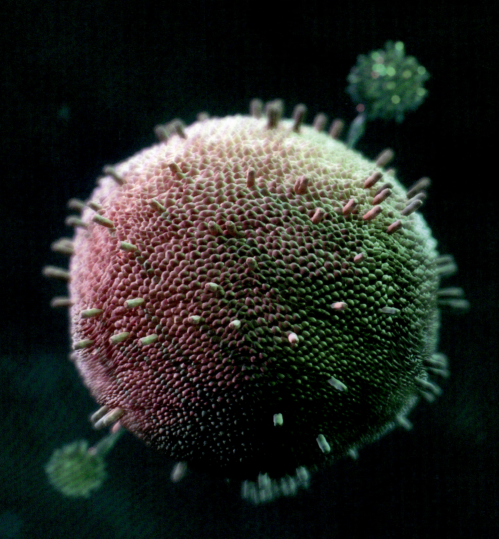

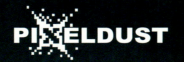

MEDICAL ANIMATION EXCELLENCE

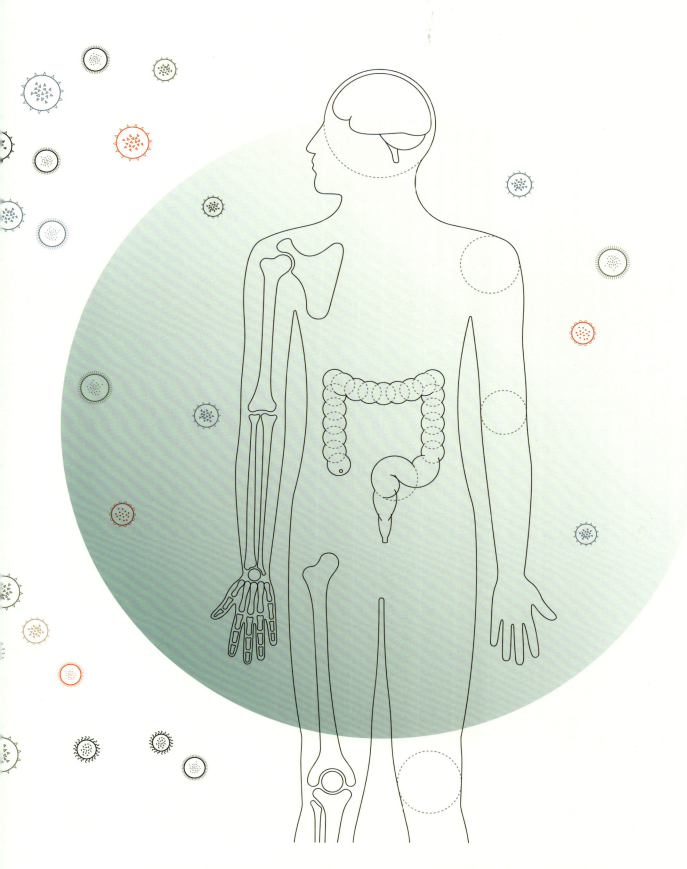

ANIMATION · DESIGN · ILLUSTRATION · VR & AR

PIXELDUST.TV

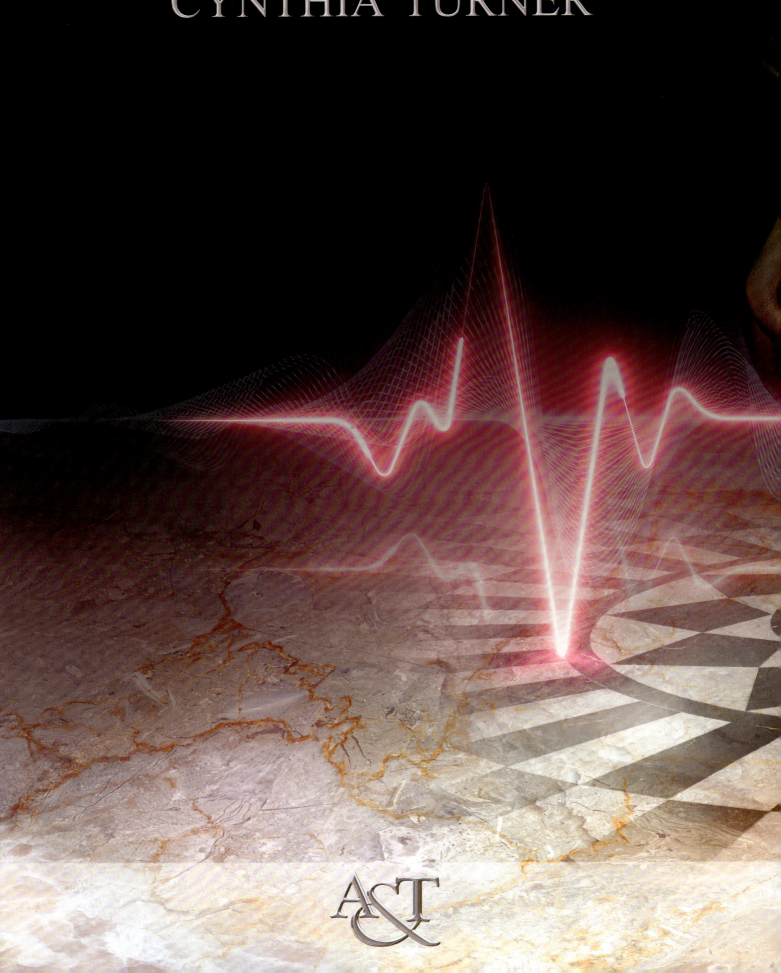

CYNTHIA TURNER

A&T

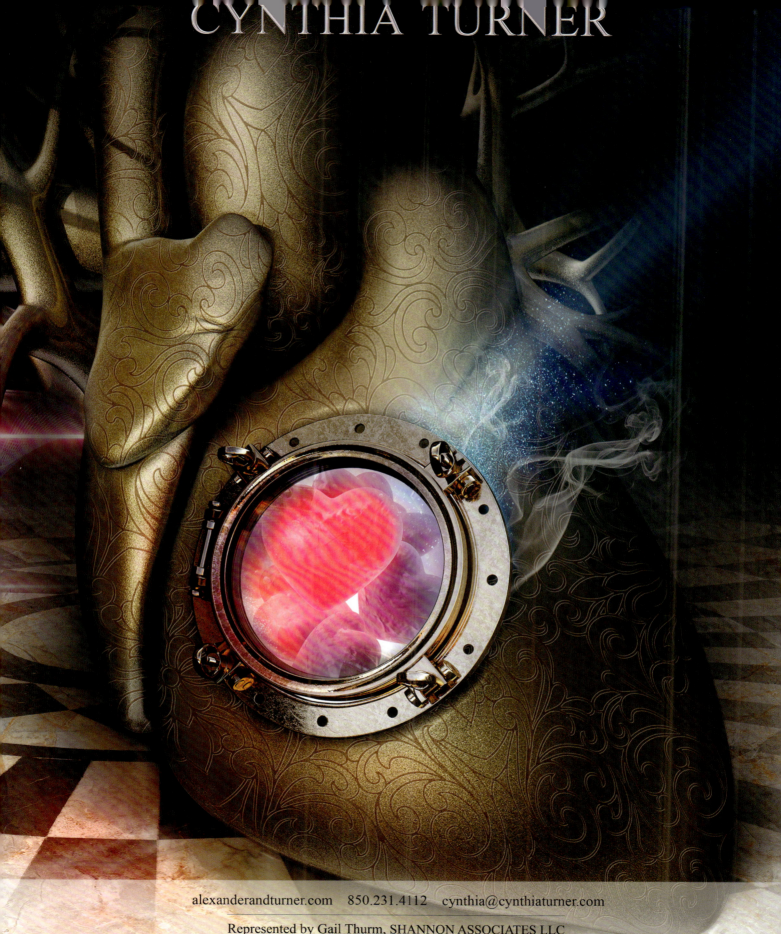

CYNTHIA TURNER

alexanderandturner.com   850.231.4112   cynthia@cynthiaturner.com

Represented by Gail Thurm, SHANNON ASSOCIATES LLC
333 W. 57th Street, Suite 809   New York, NY 10019   212.333.2551   gail@shannonassociates.com

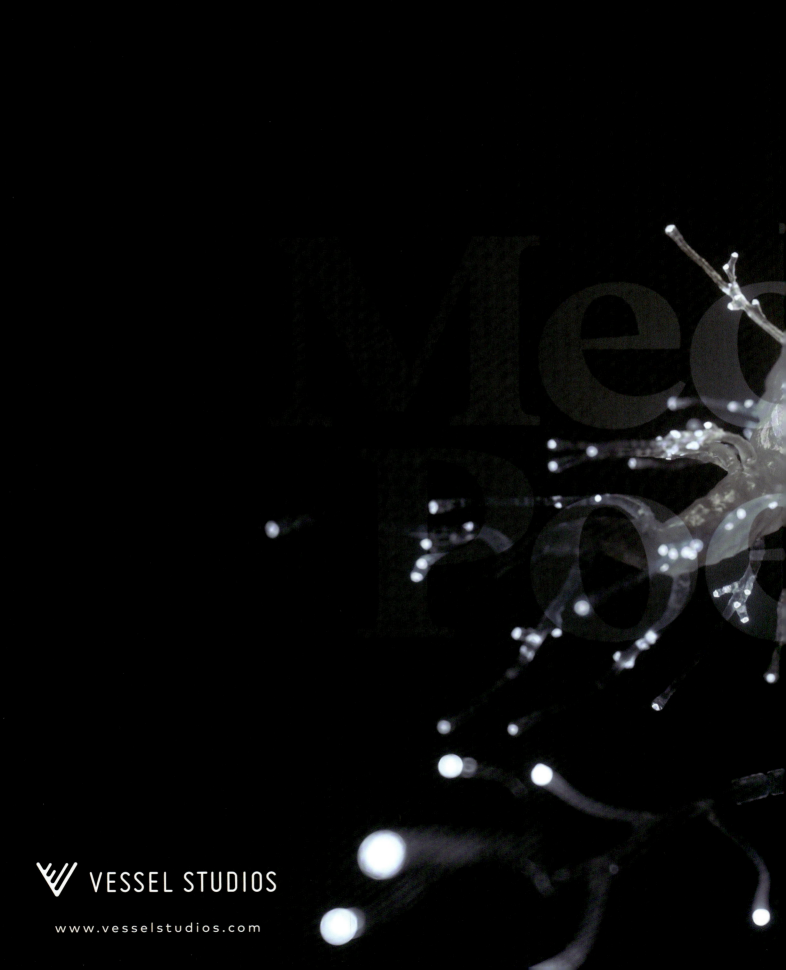

VESSEL STUDIOS

www.vesselstudios.com

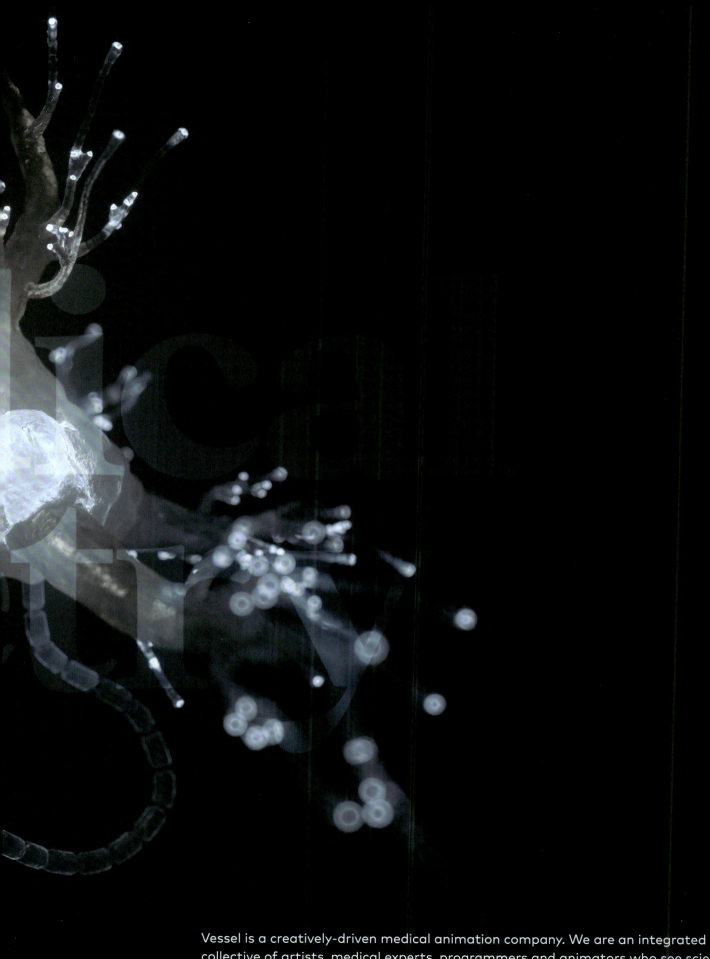

Vessel is a creatively-driven medical animation company. We are an integrated collective of artists, medical experts, programmers and animators who see science as art and narrative.

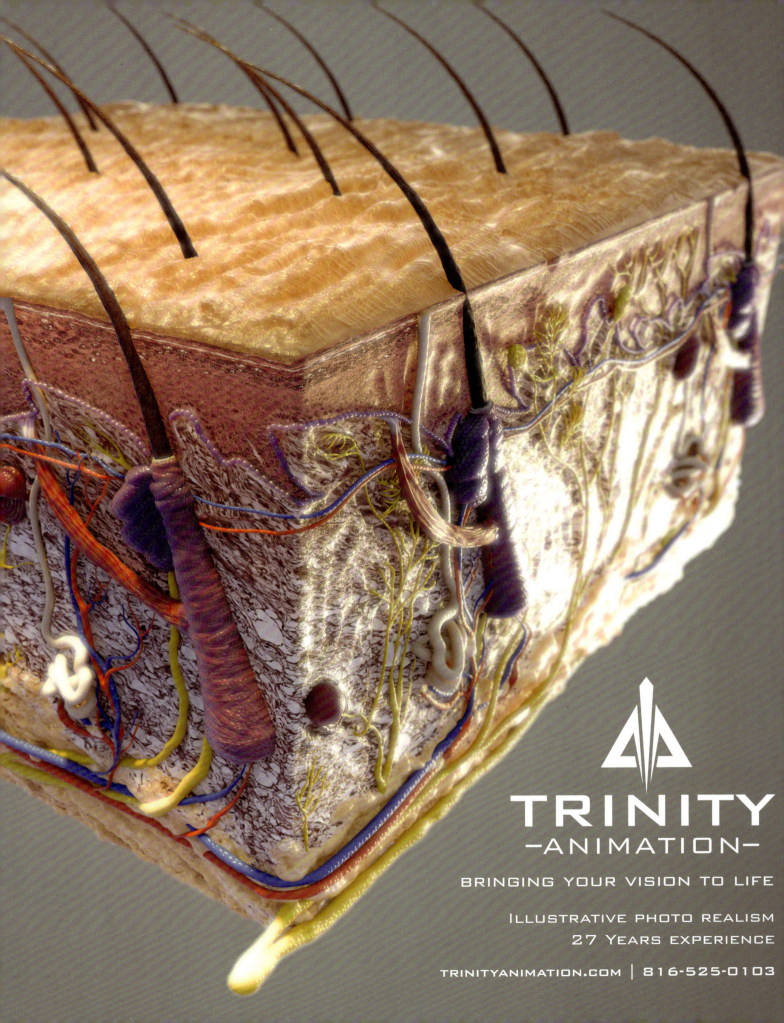

TRINITY
—ANIMATION—

BRINGING YOUR VISION TO LIFE

ILLUSTRATIVE PHOTO REALISM
27 YEARS EXPERIENCE

TRINITYANIMATION.COM | 816-525-0103

MEDICAL ILLUSTRATION

View artist portfolios online at

MEDILLSB.COM

View artist portfolios online at

MEDILLSB.COM

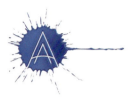

Big AI Gruswitz

AAA Rep. Unipessoal Lda
www.aaarep.net
antonio@aaarep.net
Tel: +351-910358405

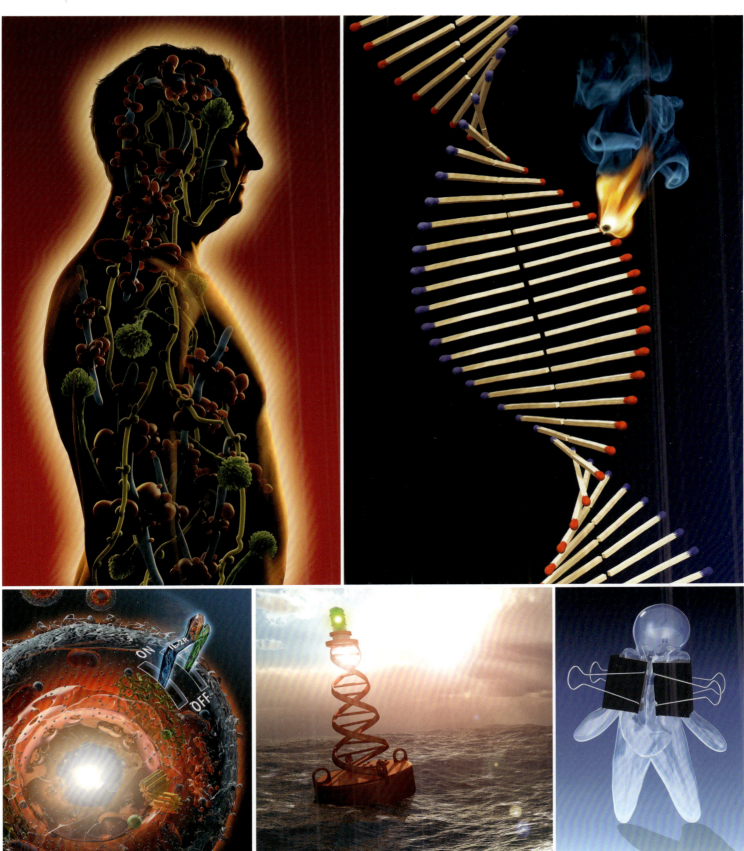

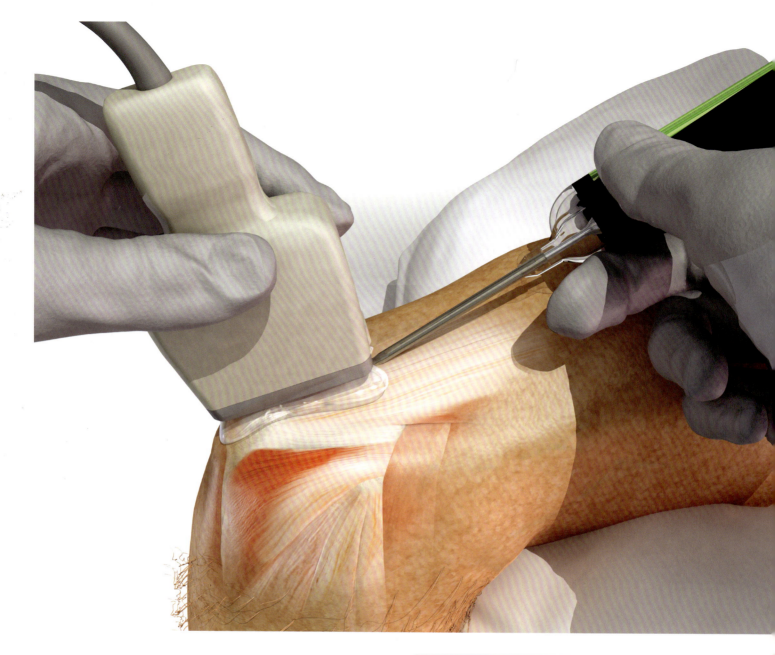

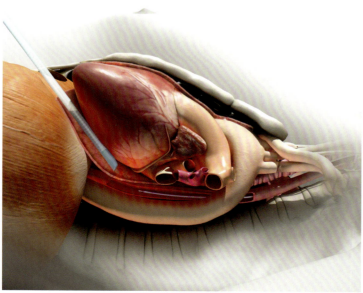

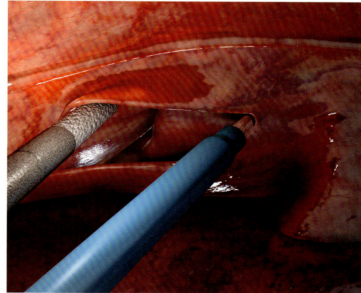

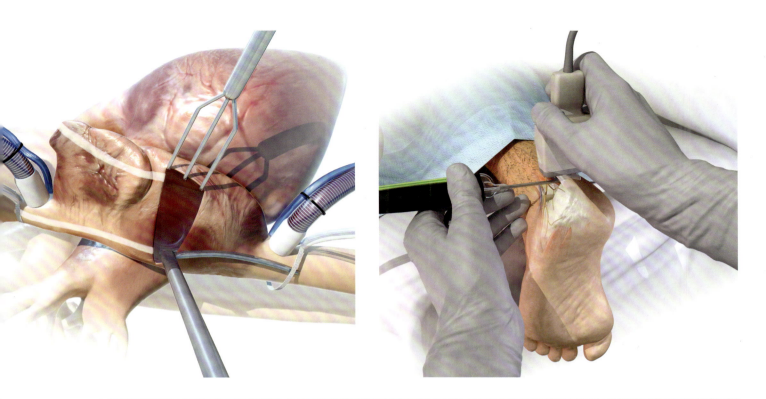

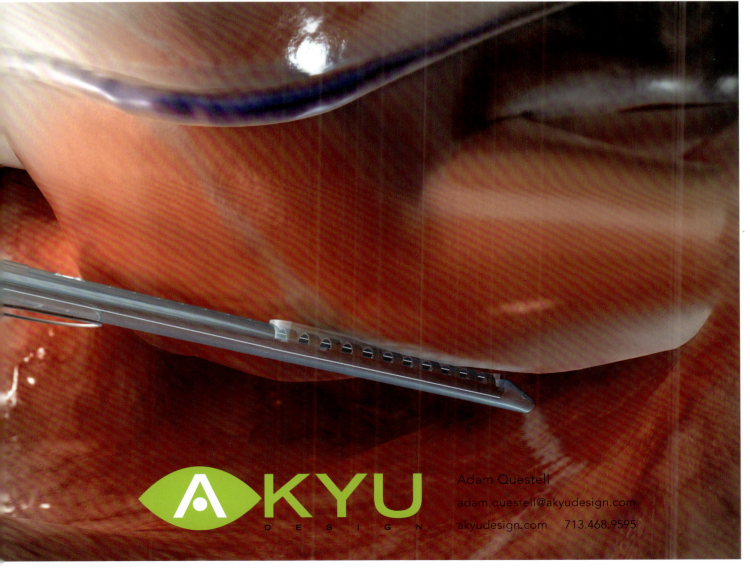

Adam Questell
adam.questell@akyudesign.com
akyudesign.com   713.468.9595

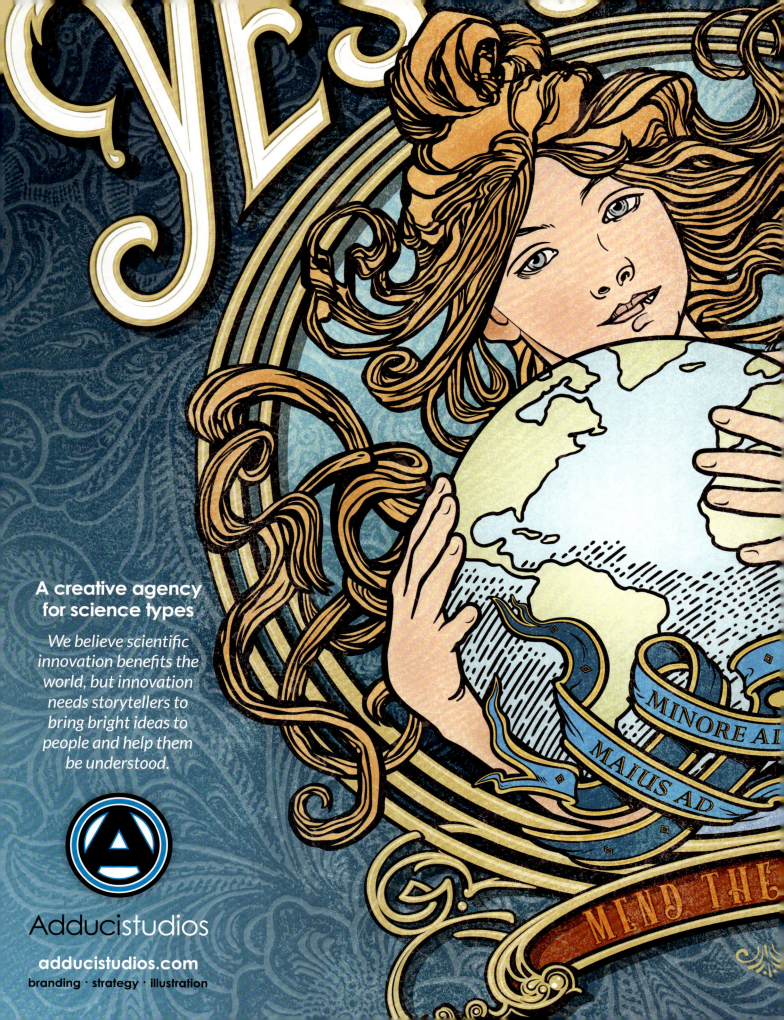

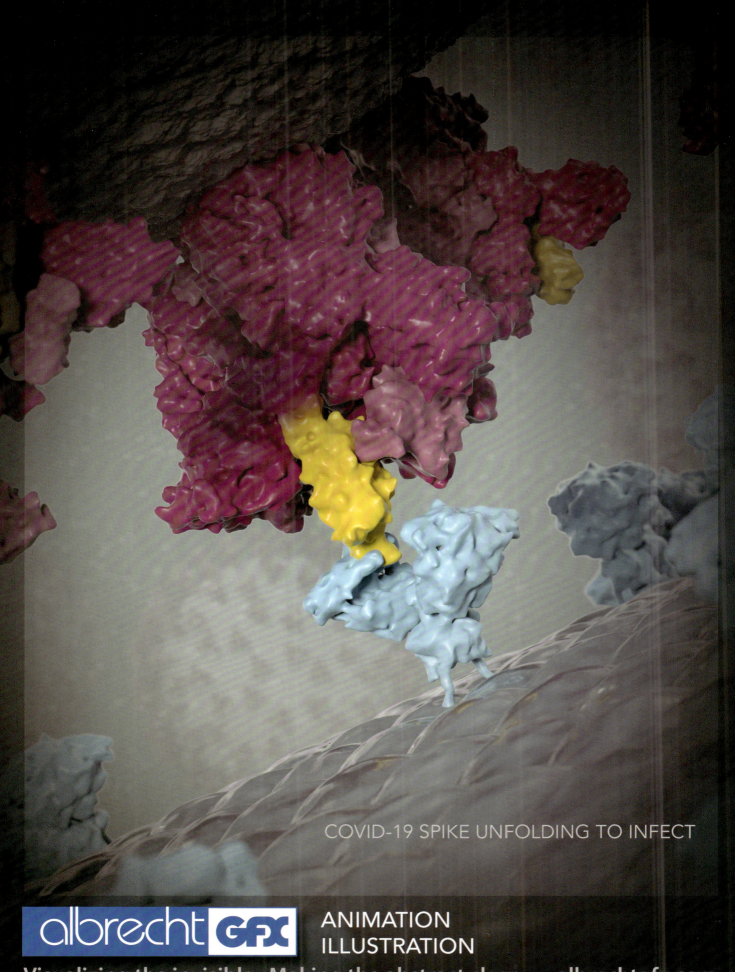

COVID-19 SPIKE UNFOLDING TO INFECT

albrecht GFX
ANIMATION
ILLUSTRATION
Visualizing the invisible. Making the abstract clear. • albrechtgfx.com

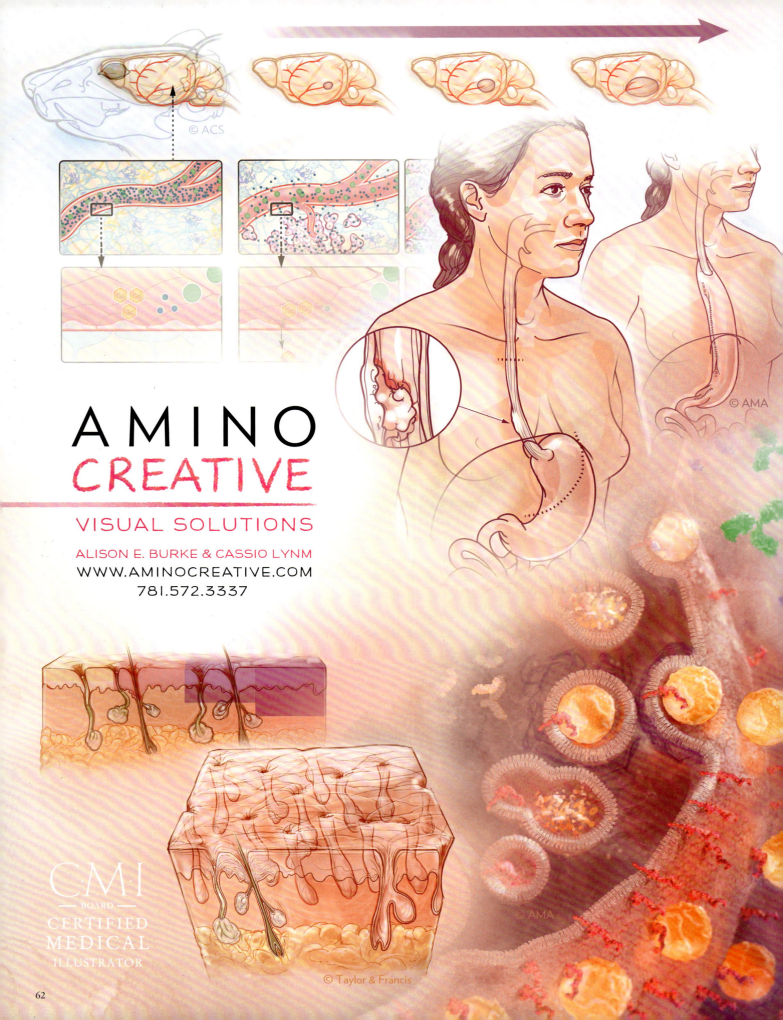

© ACS

© AMA

© AMA

© Taylor & Francis

AMINO
CREATIVE

VISUAL SOLUTIONS

ALISON E. BURKE & CASSIO LYNM

WWW.AMINOCREATIVE.COM
781.572.3337

CMI
BOARD

CERTIFIED
MEDICAL
ILLUSTRATOR

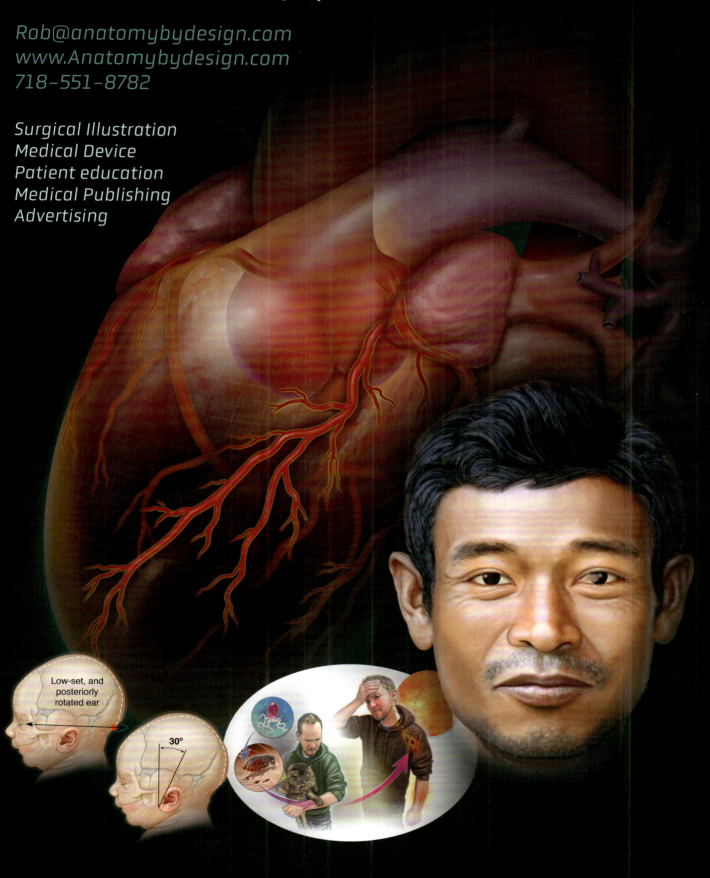

Anatomy By Design, Inc.

Rob@anatomybydesign.com
www.Anatomybydesign.com
718-551-8782

Surgical Illustration
Medical Device
Patient education
Medical Publishing
Advertising

Low-set, and posteriorly rotated ear

30°

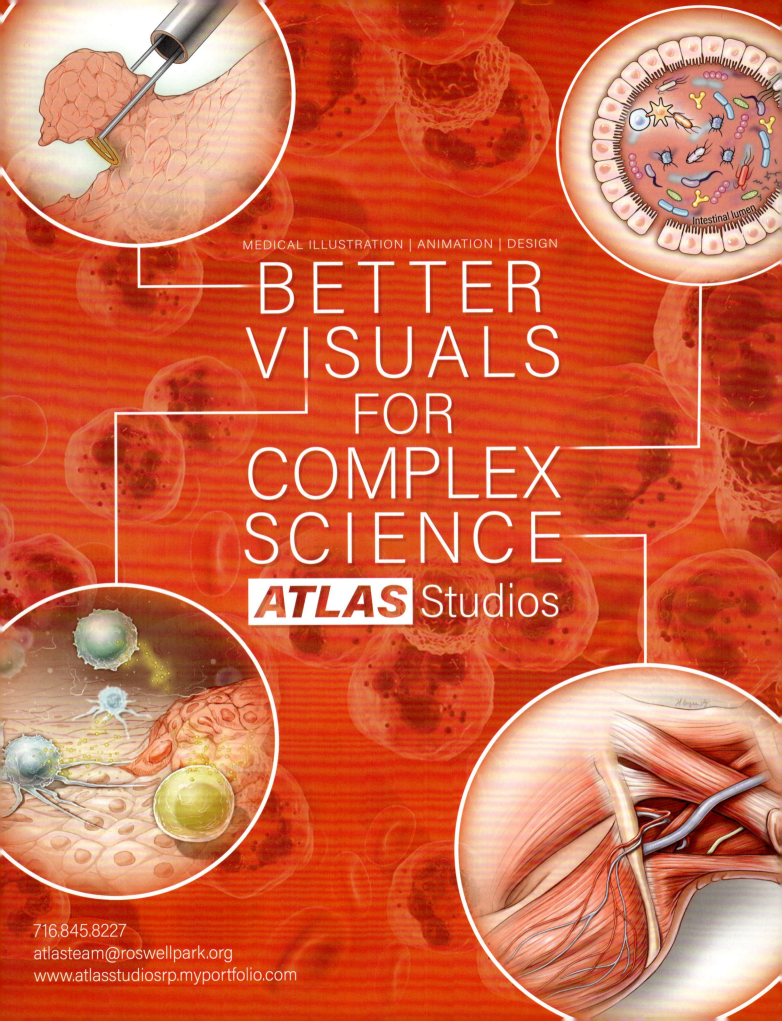

MEDICAL ILLUSTRATION | ANIMATION | DESIGN

BETTER VISUALS FOR COMPLEX SCIENCE

ATLAS Studios

Intestinal lumen

716.845.8227
atlasteam@roswellpark.org
www.atlasstudiosrp.myportfolio.com

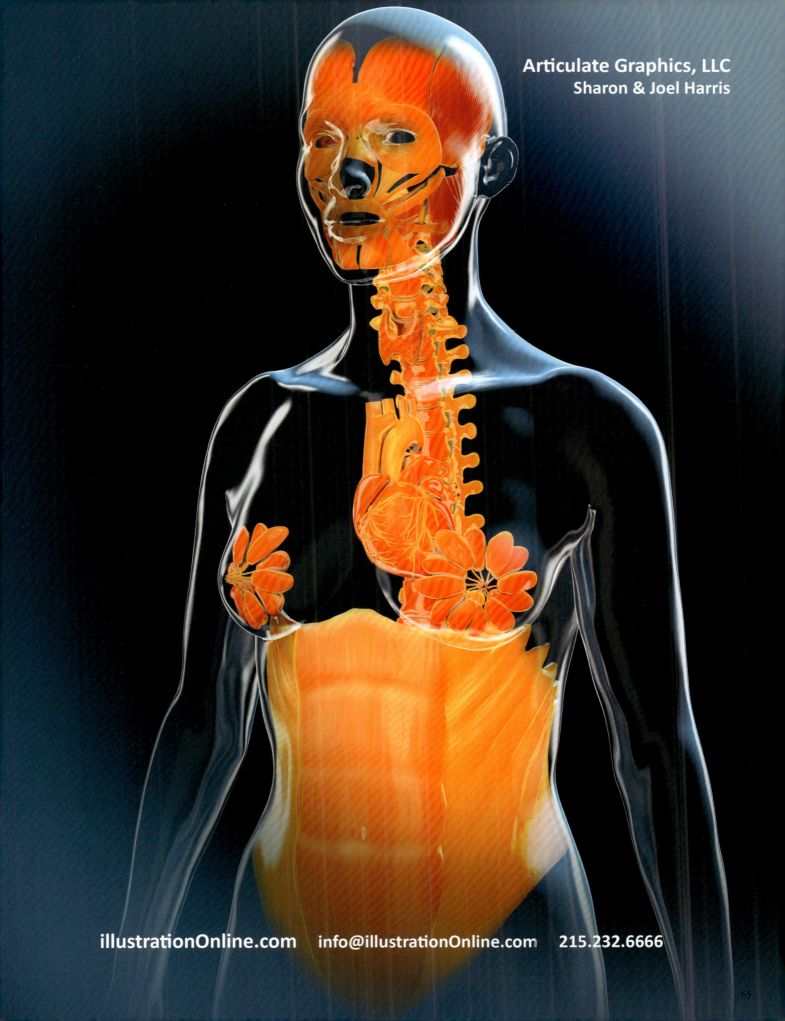

Articulate Graphics, LLC
Sharon & Joel Harris

illustrationOnline.com   info@illustrationOnline.com   215.232.6666

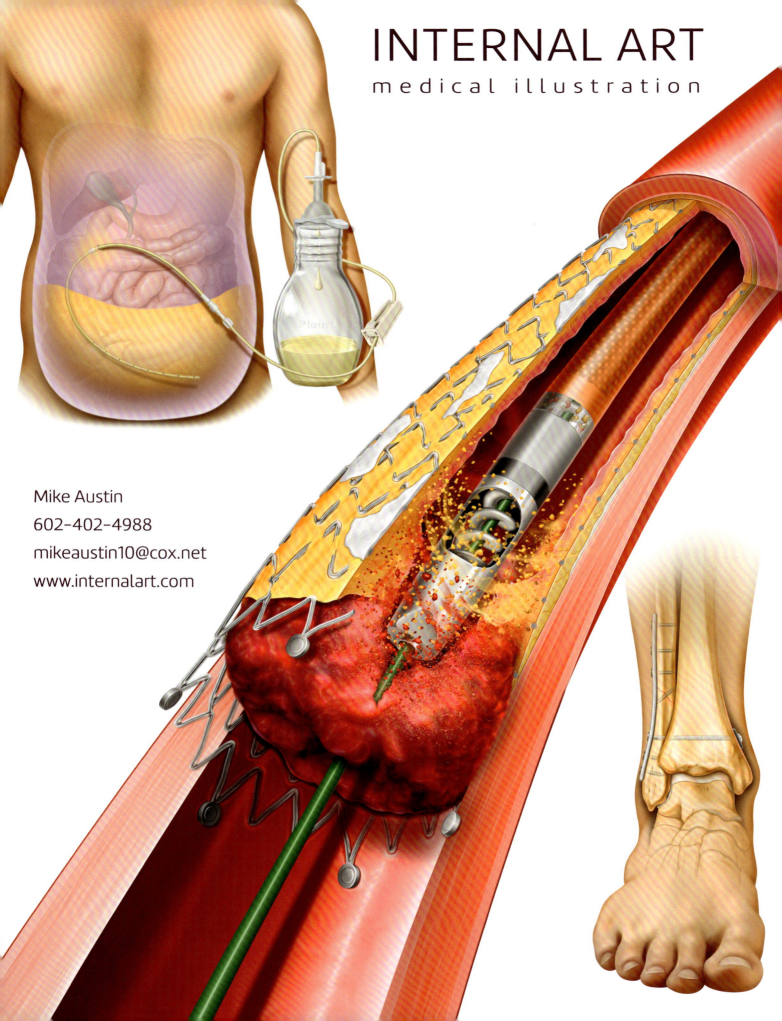

INTERNAL ART
medical illustration

Mike Austin

602-402-4988

mikeaustin10@cox.net

www.internalart.com

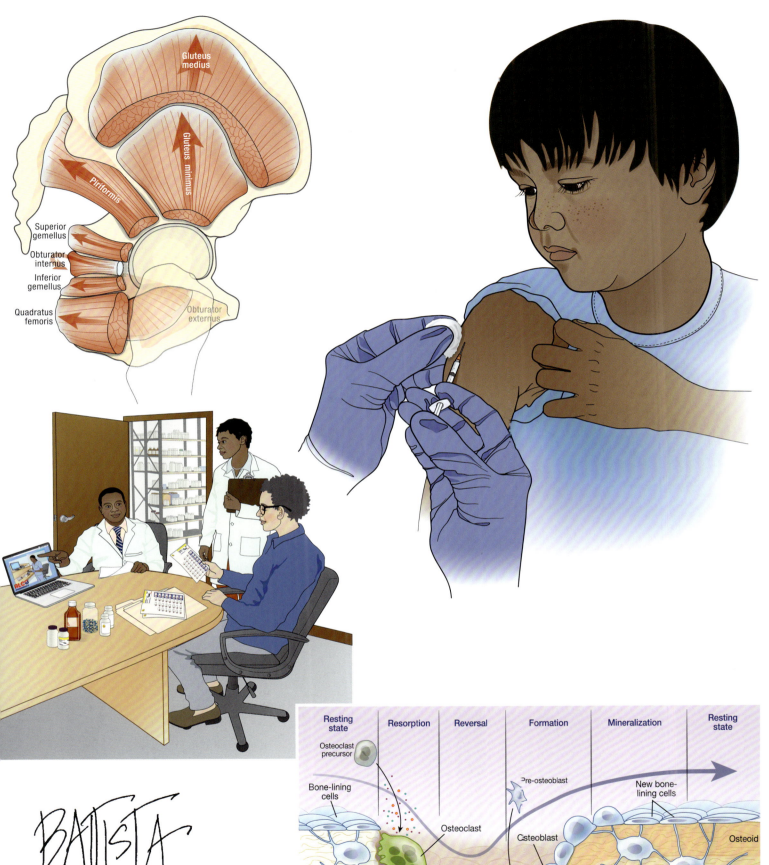

Gluteus medius

Gluteus minimus

Piriformis

Superior gemellus

Obturator internus

Inferior gemellus

Quadratus femoris

Obturator externus

ALCO

BATTISTA

Kimberly Battista
2123 Bank Street
Baltimore, Maryland 21231
410.428.2782

www.battistaillustration.com

Resting state	Resorption	Reversal	Formation	Mineralization	Resting state

Osteoclast precursor

Bone-lining cells

Pre-osteoblast

New bone-lining cells

Osteoclast

Osteoblast

Osteoid

New bone

Macrophages

Cement line

Osteocytes

Old bone

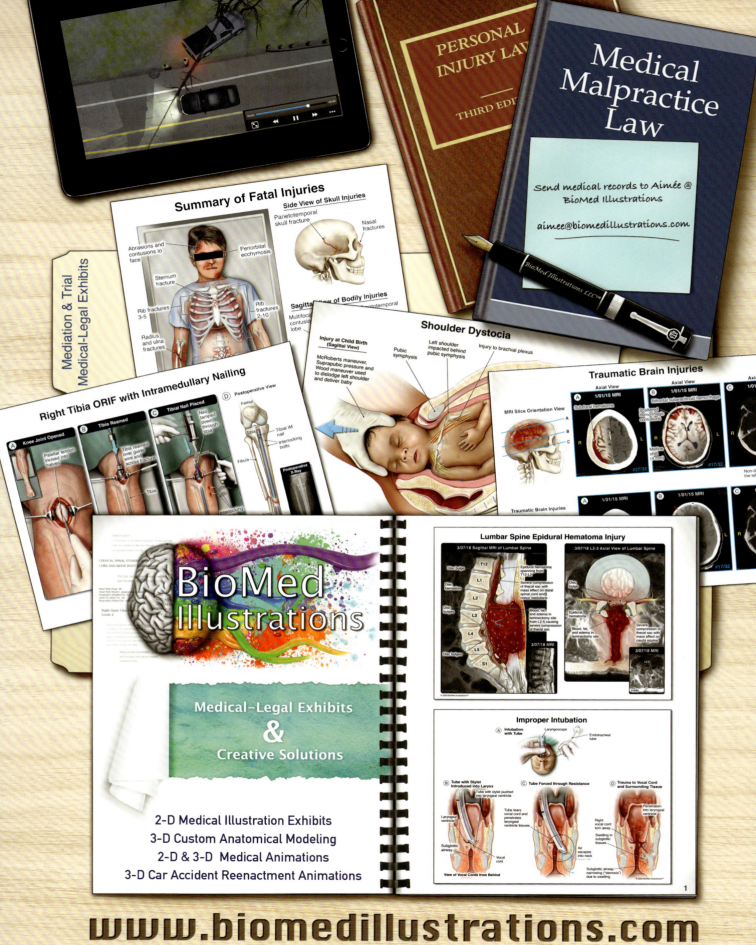

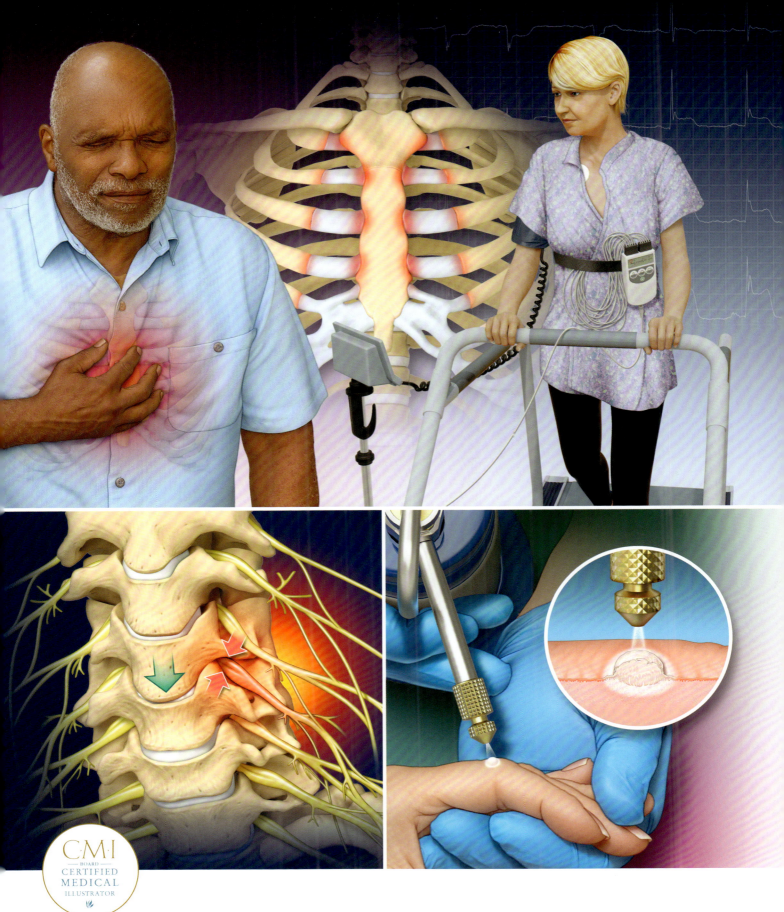

CMI
BOARD
CERTIFIED
MEDICAL
ILLUSTRATOR

BioMedical Art

John W. Karapelou, CMI • www.biomedicalart.com • info@biomedicalart.com • 216.291.6050

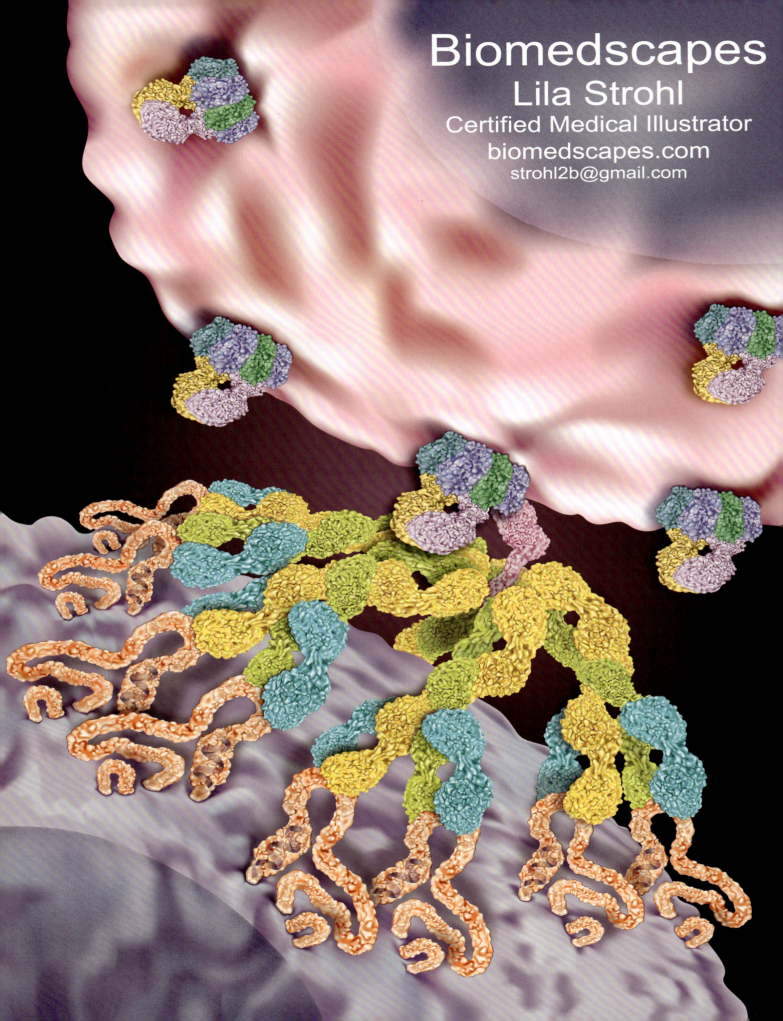

Biomedscapes
Lila Strohl
Certified Medical Illustrator
biomedscapes.com
strohl2b@gmail.com

Bodell Medical Media

scott@bodellmedia.com

214-695-9086

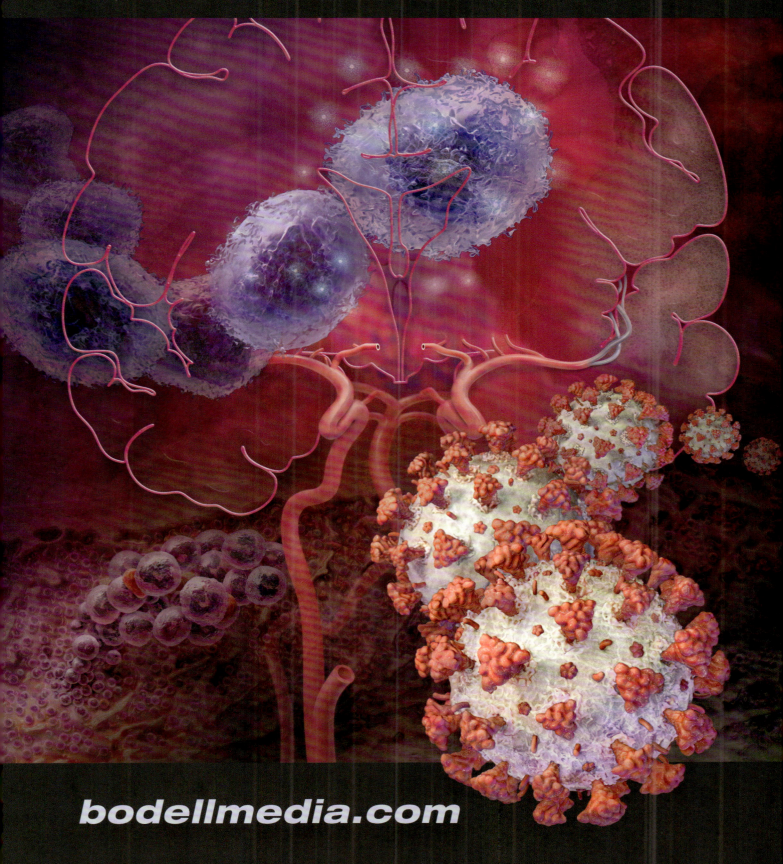

bodellmedia.com

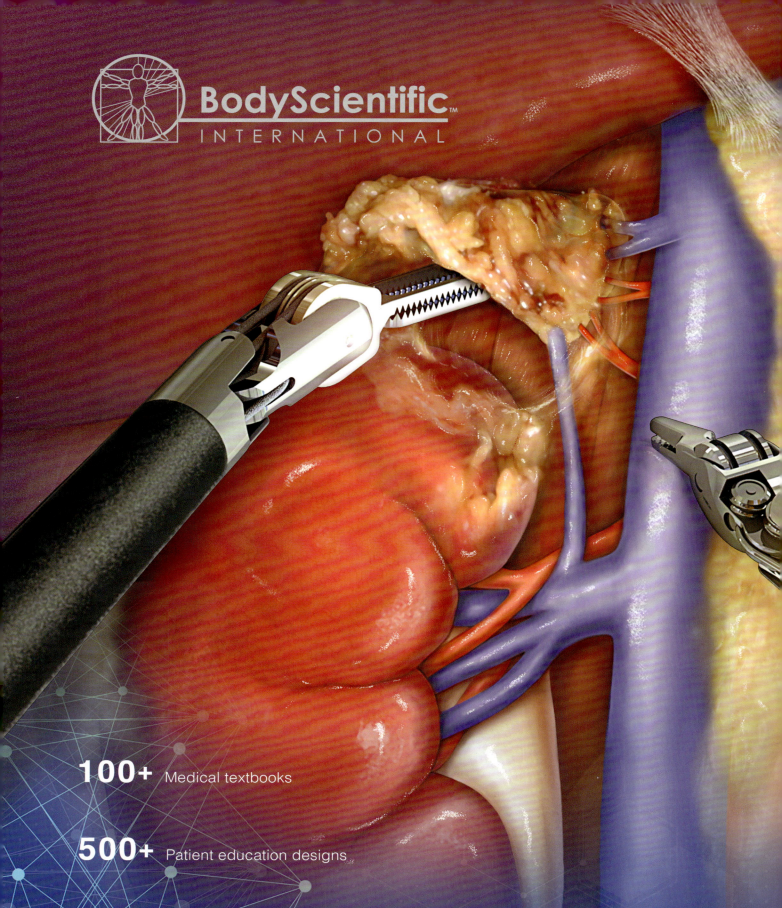

BodyScientific™

INTERNATIONAL

100+ Medical textbooks

500+ Patient education designs

5,000+ Medical images for licensing

© 2021 Body Scientific International, LLC

72

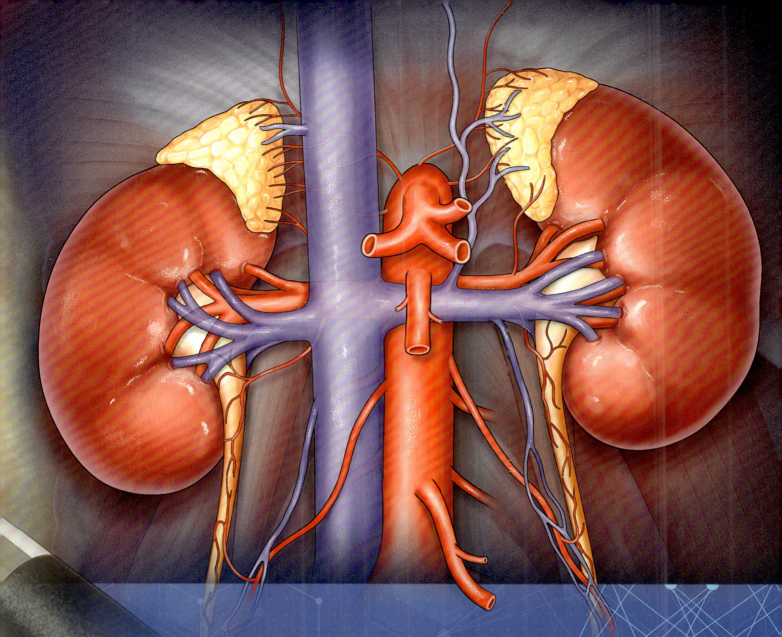

High fidelity medical designs for:
- Medical publishers
- Pharmaceutical
- Medical device
- Medical training solutions
- Online patient education
- Healthcare associations

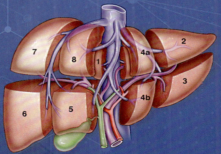

Services:

Illustration & Animation | Anatomical Models |
Patient Education Products | Virtual Technology Solutions

Body Scientific International
www.BodyScientific.com
info@bodyscientific.com
1 833 263 9724

Follow us

© 2021 Body Scientific International, LLC

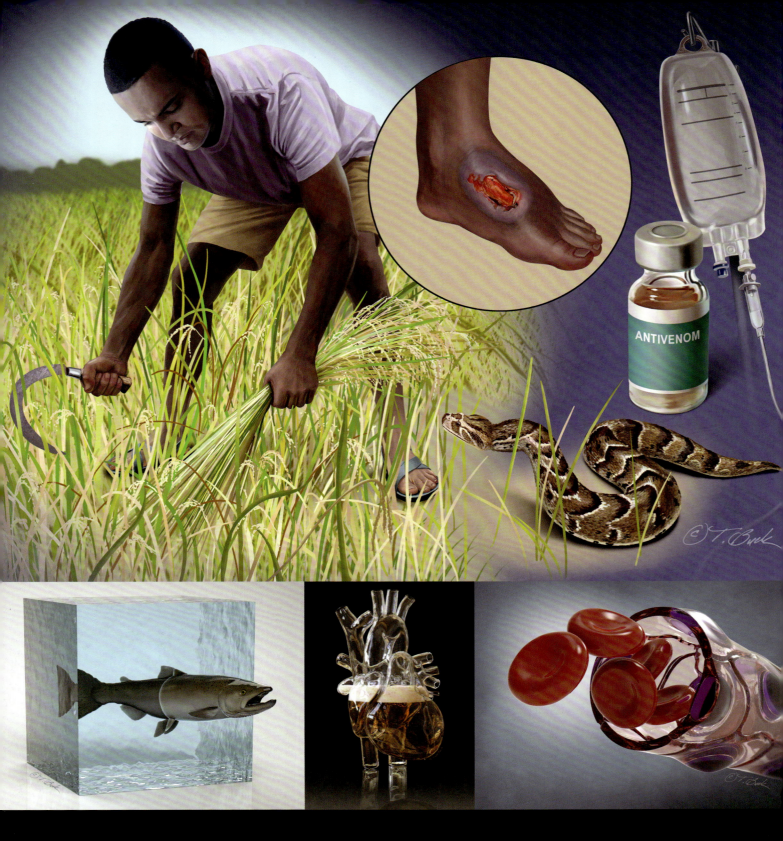

Todd Buck Illustration LLC   buckart@earthlink.net   www.todbuck.com   630 627 0903

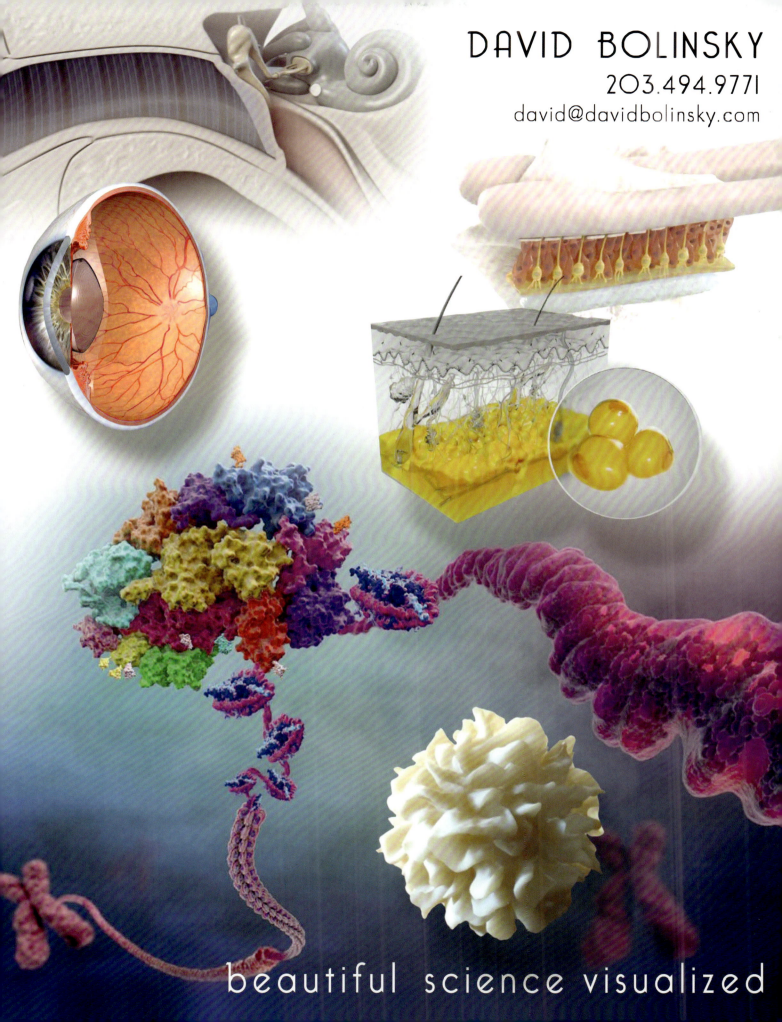

DAVID BOLINSKY

203.494.9771

david@davidbolinsky.com

beautiful science visualized

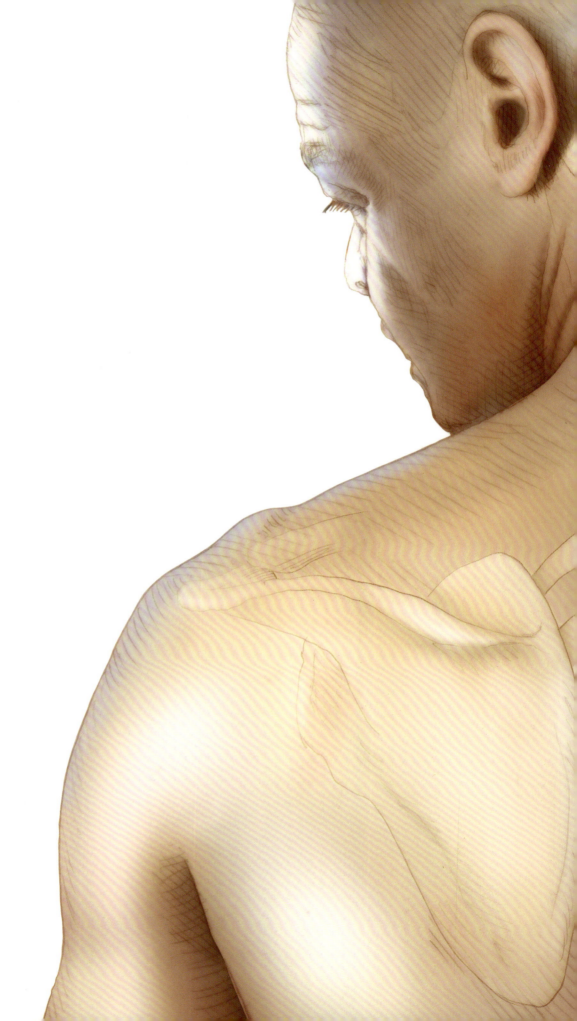

MOLLY BORMAN

Illustrating the Science of Anatomy

www.mborman.com

970 420 8136

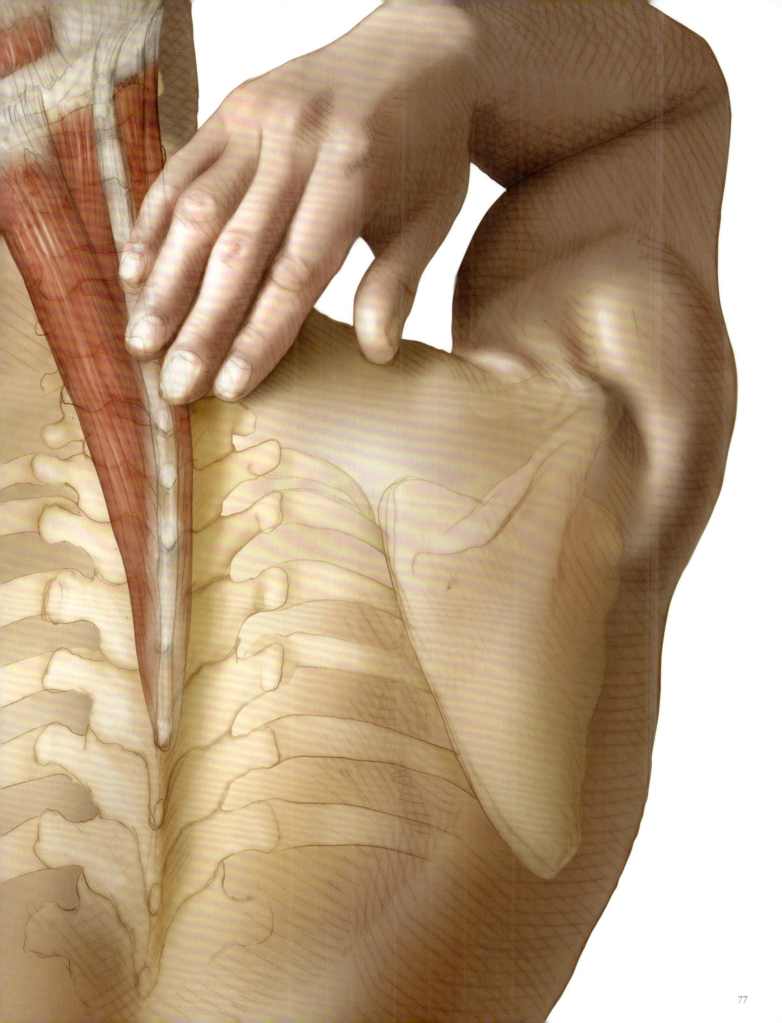

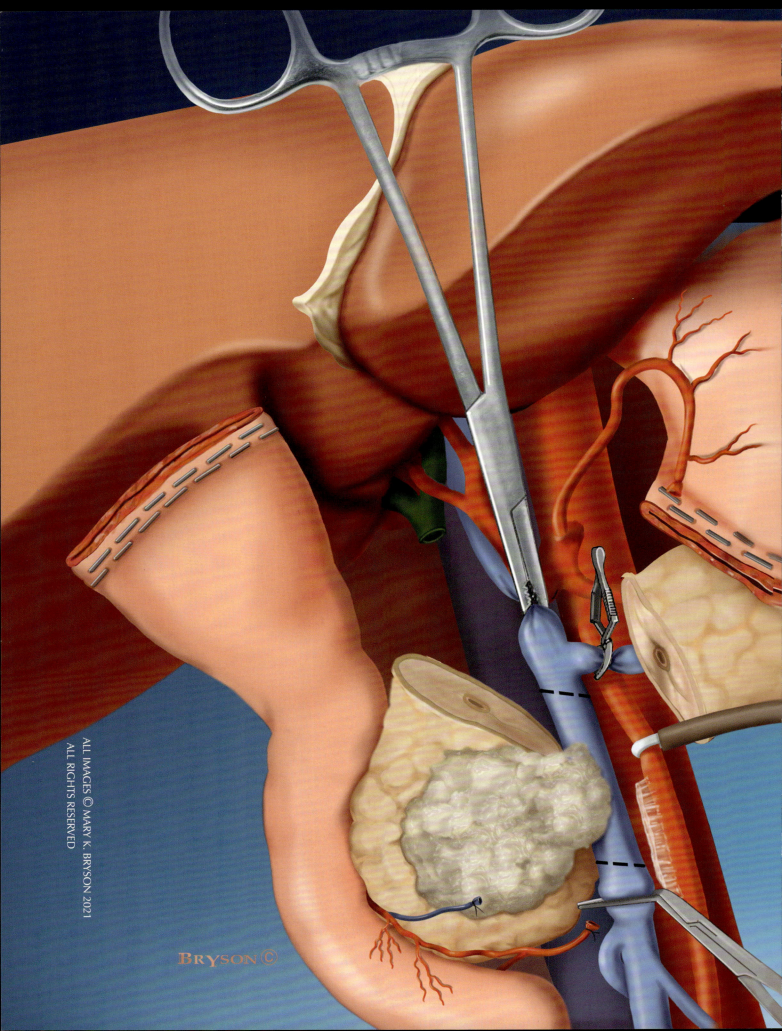

ALL IMAGES © MARY K. BRYSON 2021
ALL RIGHTS RESERVED

BRYSON ©

brysonbiomed.com

Mary K. Bryson, M.A.M.S.
mary@brysonbiomed.com

610 517-3298

 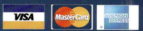

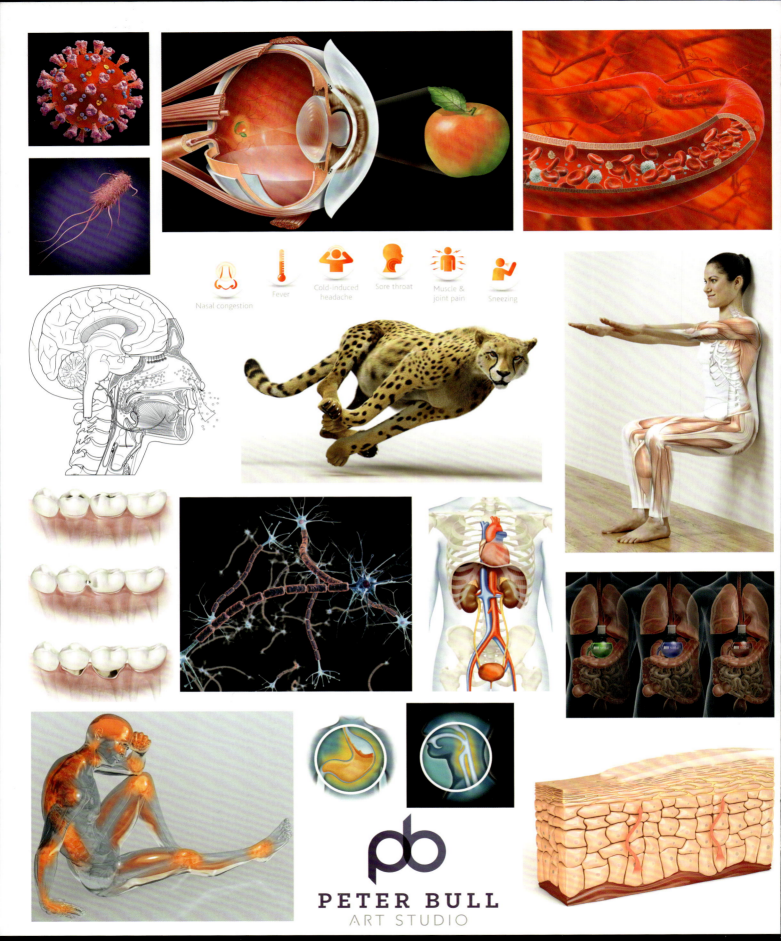

PETER BULL
ART STUDIO

Medical, Science & Natural History illustration and animation

01144 1892 890296 • peter@peterbullartstudio.co.uk • www.peterbullartstudio.co.uk

Nasal congestion

Fever

Cold-induced headache

Sore throat

Muscle & joint pain

Sneezing

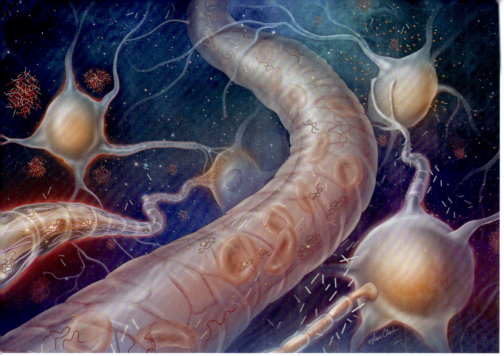
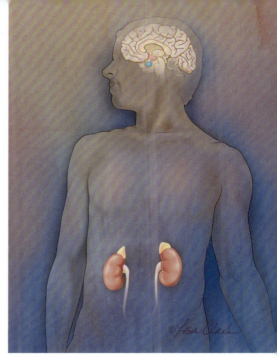
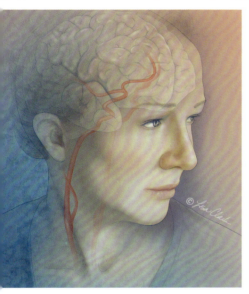

![Clark Illustration logo]

clark
illustration

www.clark-illustration.com
214.284.5974
info@clark-illustration.com

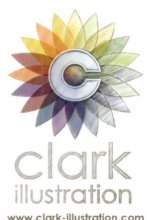
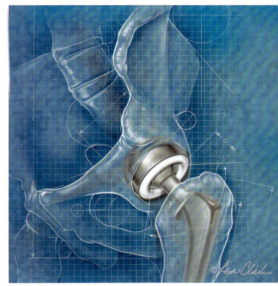
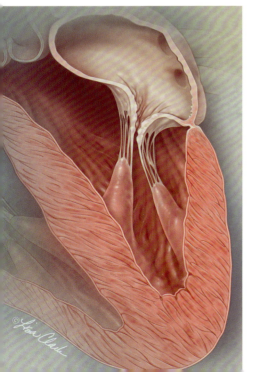
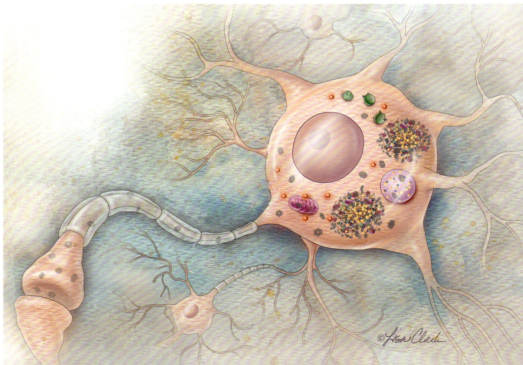

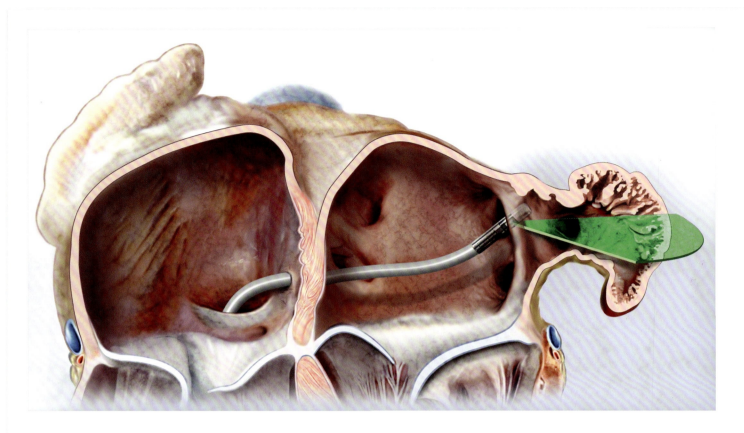

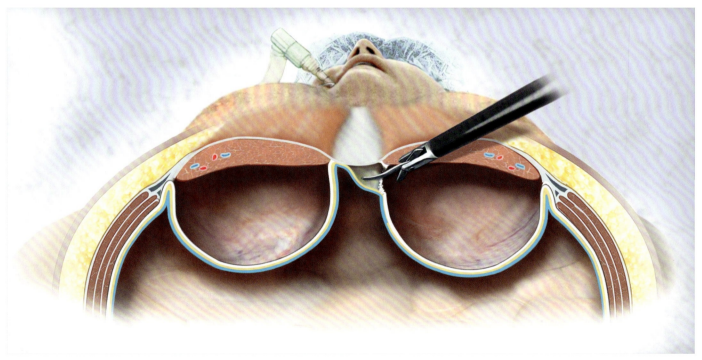

Chovan
Healthcare Visuals, LLC
joechovan@icloud.com

513.312.1394

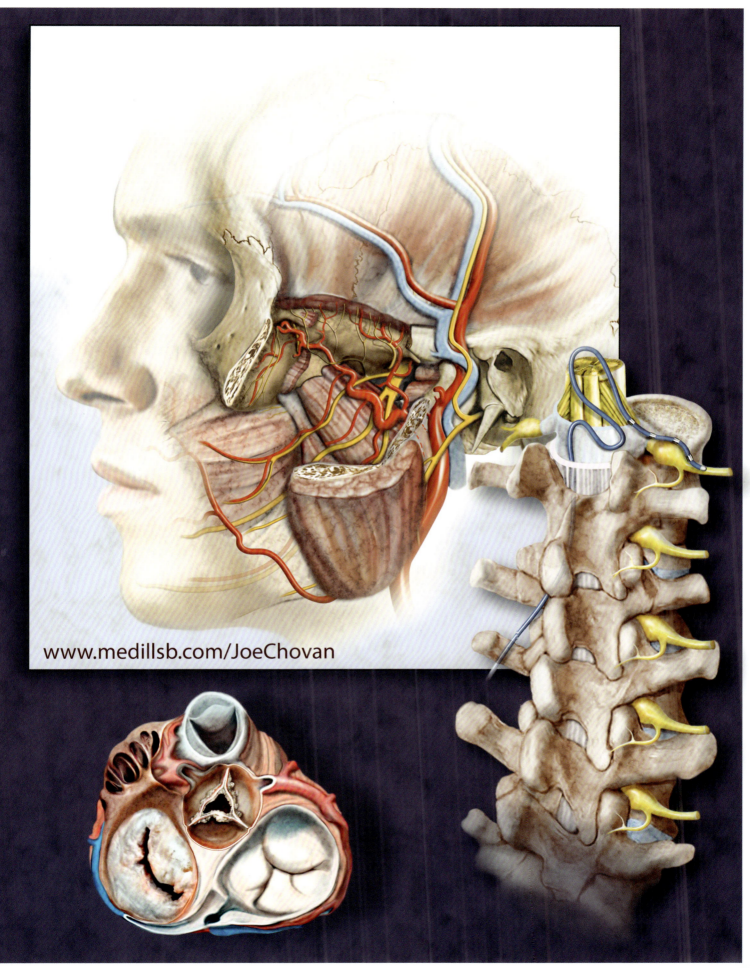

www.medillsb.com/JoeChovan

Cooley Studios

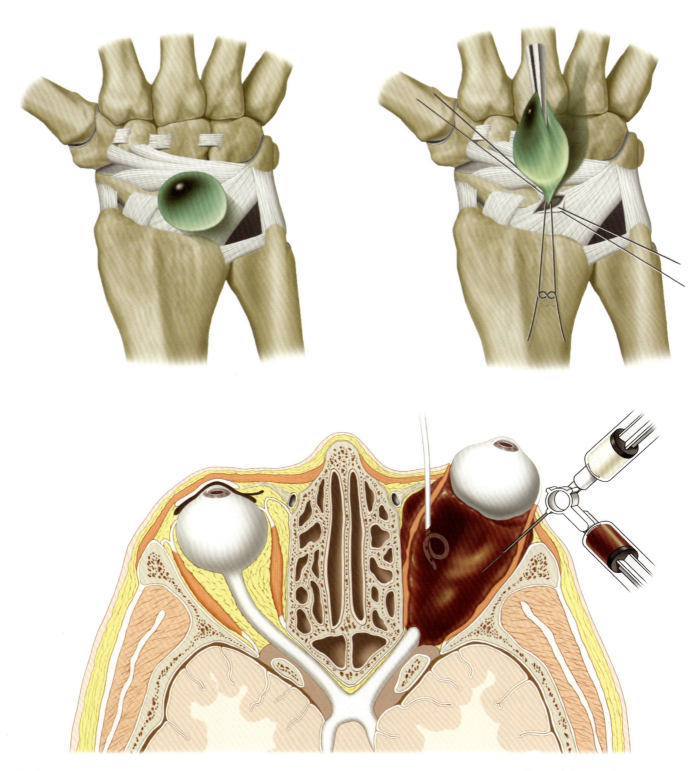

All artwork © M. Cooley

Michael A. Cooley, MFA
Cooley Studios
870 North High Street, Suite 11/ Worthington, Ohio 43085
cooleystudios.com/ info@cooleystudios.com/ 614-547-7900

Marie Dauenheimer, MA, CMI, FAMI
Medical Visualization and Animation

dauenheimer@rcn.com   mariedauenheimer.com   571.216.1472

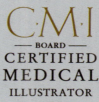

CMI
— BOARD —
CERTIFIED
MEDICAL
ILLUSTRATOR

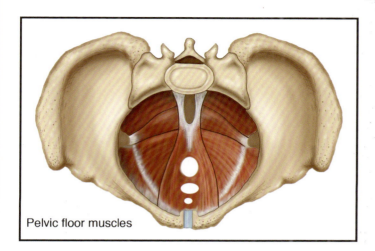

Pelvic floor muscles

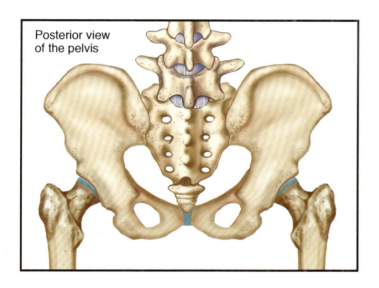

Posterior view
of the pelvis

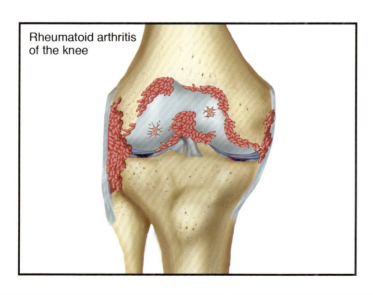

Rheumatoid arthritis
of the knee

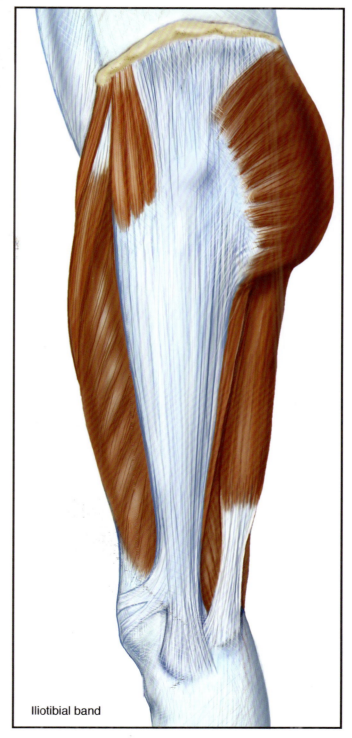

Iliotibial band

Representing 170 highly selected illustrators and motion artists, many of whom have a strong area of specialty and considerable experience working on life sciences related material.

Selected artists' portfolios are available to review by searching 'By Name' for 'Debut Art' on http://www.medillsb.com

Début Art has offices in London and New York with an experienced and talented team to help regarding enquiries.

The whole team can be contacted via email sent to info@debutart.com One of the team will respond to your enquiry promptly.

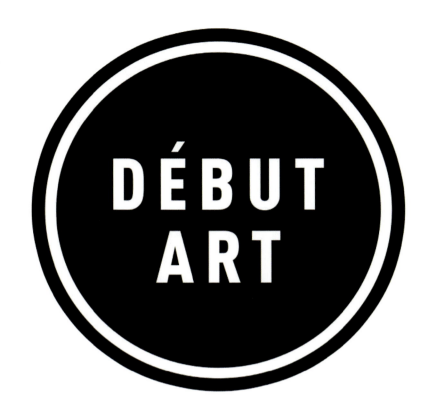

Est. 1985

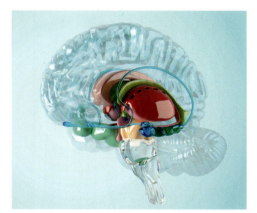

Comm. for Runner's World Magazine

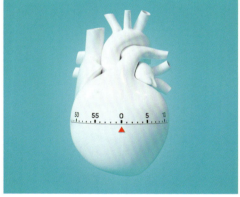

Comm. for University of Miami

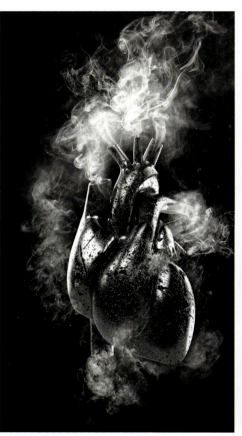

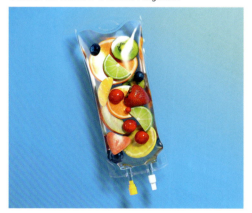

Comm. for Women's Health Magazine

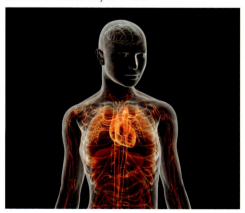

Comm. for Wall Street Journal

Comm. for Sinai Hospital

Début Art • Illustrators, Motion Artists & Illustrative Designers Agents.
420 West 14th Street, Suite 5SW, NY 10014. Tel: 212 995 5044
30 Tottenham Street, London, W1T 4RJ. United Kingdom. Tel: 01144 20 7636 1064

email: **info@debutart.com** • **www.debutart.com** • **@debutart**

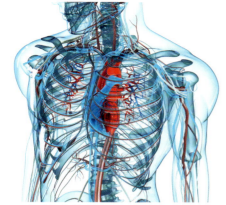
Comm. for Men's Health Magazine

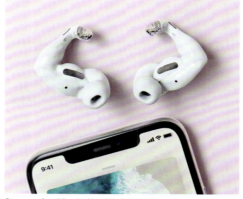
Comm. for Men's Health Magazine

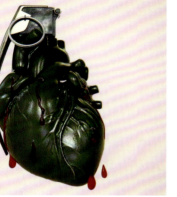
Comm. for Men's Health Magazine

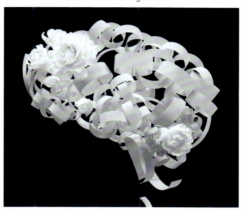
Comm. for a Global Management Consultancy

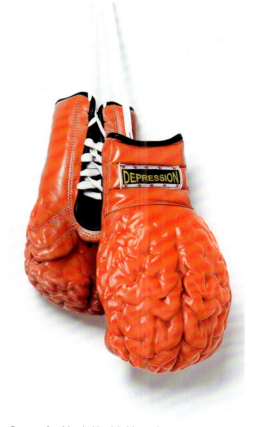
Comm. for Men's Health Magazine

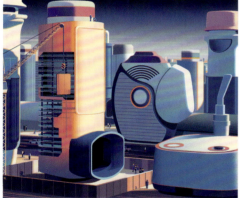
Comm. for Nature Outlook

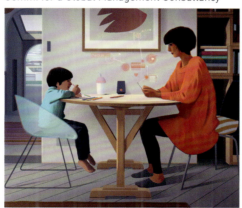
Comm. for Deloitte

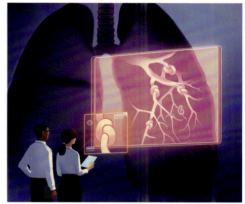
Comm. for Nature Outlook

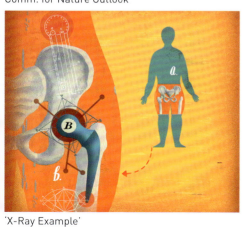
'X-Ray Example'

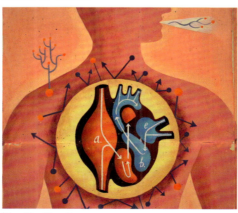
'Healthy Heart'

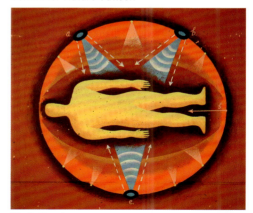
'Body Scan'

Début Art • Illustrators, Motion Artists & Illustrative Designers Agents.
420 West 14th Street, Suite 5SW, NY 10014. Tel: 212 995 5044
30 Tottenham Street, London, W1T 4RJ. United Kingdom. Tel: 01144 20 7636 1064

email: **info@debutart.com** • **www.debutart.com** • **@debutart**

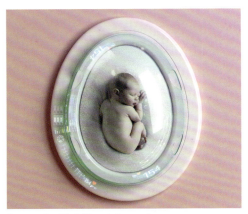

Comm. for Wall Street Journal

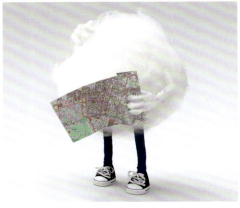

Comm. for Langland

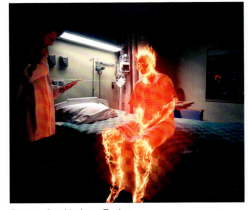

Comm. for Abelson Taylor

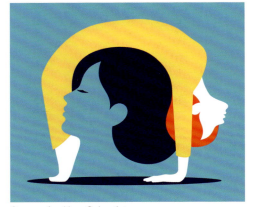

Comm. for New Scientist

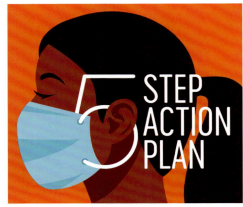

Comm. for Supermarket News

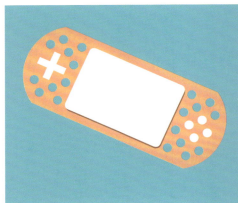

Comm. for New Scientist

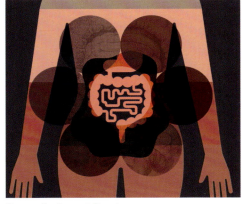

Comm. for Lancet Oncology

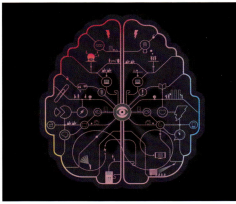

Comm. for IEEE Magazine

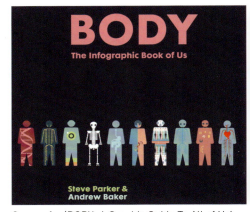

Comm. for 'BODY: A Graphic Guide To All of Us'

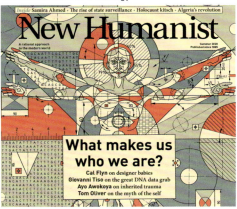

Comm. for New Scientist

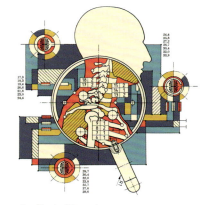

Comm. for Proto Magazine

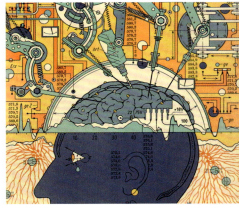

Comm. for Psychologie Heute

Début Art • Illustrators, Motion Artists & Illustrative Designers Agents.
420 West 14th Street, Suite 5SW, NY 10014. Tel: 212 995 5044
30 Tottenham Street, London, W1T 4RJ. United Kingdom. Tel: 01144 20 7636 1064

email: **info@debutart.com** • **www.debutart.com** • **@debutart**

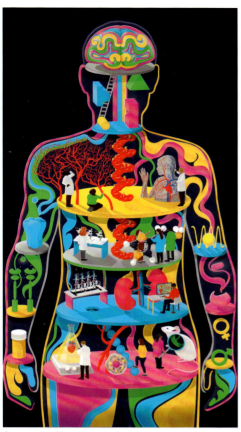

Comm. for The Watts Lab

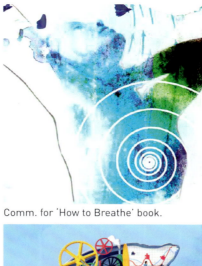

Comm. for 'How to Breathe' book.

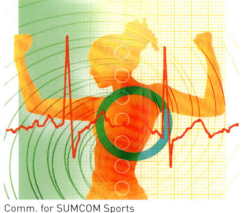

Comm. for SUMCOM Sports

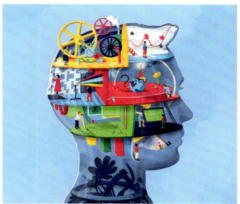

Comm. for The Guardian

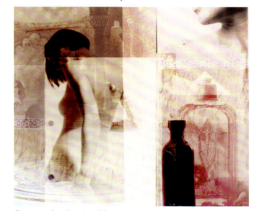

Comm. for Lactacid

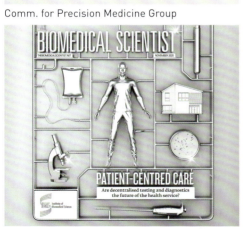

Comm. for Precision Medicine Group

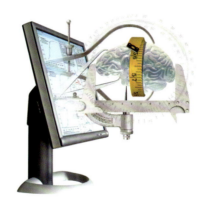

'Big Data'

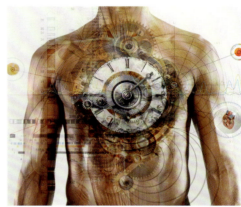

Comm. for Popular Science Magazine

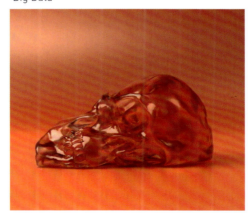

Comm. for Biomedical Scientist

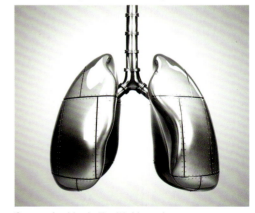

'Jelly Skull'

Comm. for Men's Health Magazine

Début Art • Illustrators, Motion Artists & Illustrative Designers Agents.
420 West 14th Street, Suite 5SW, NY 10014. Tel: 212 995 5044
30 Tottenham Street, London, W1T 4RJ. United Kingdom. Tel: 01144 20 7636 1064

email: **info@debutart.com** • **www.debutart.com** • **@debutart**

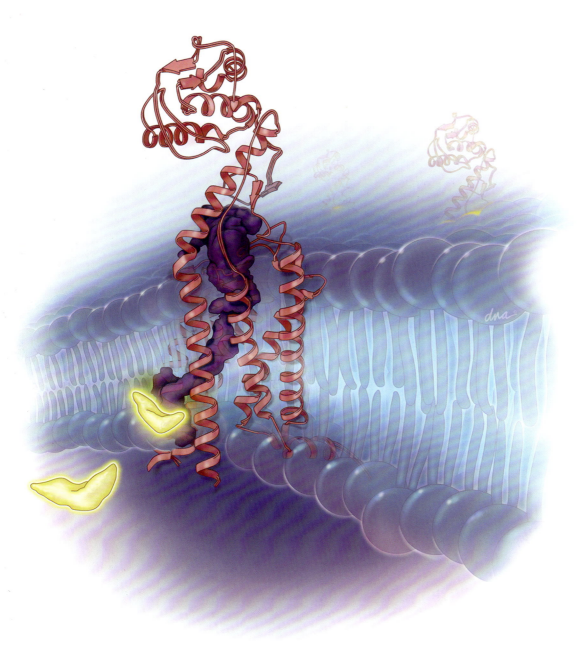

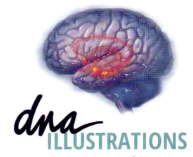

dna
ILLUSTRATIONS

Anatomy and Surgery
Editorial Illustration
Mechanism of Action
Patient Education
Immunology
Maternal/Fetal Medicine

alex@dnaillustrations.com
www.**dna**illustrations.com

Inventive solutions. Accurate results.

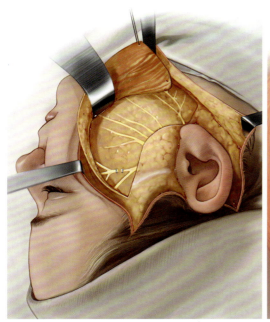

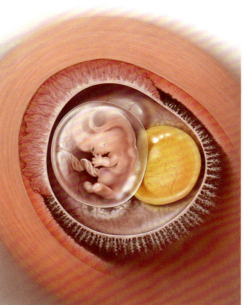

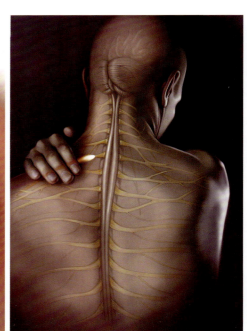

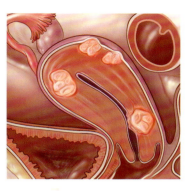

A resource
for **medical**
& biological
illustration

C·M·I
BOARD
CERTIFIED
MEDICAL
ILLUSTRATOR

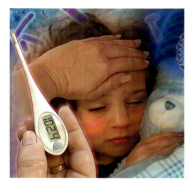

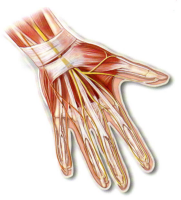

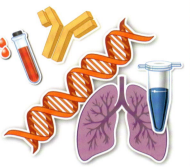

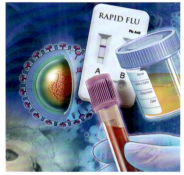

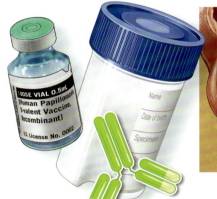

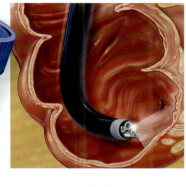

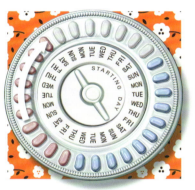

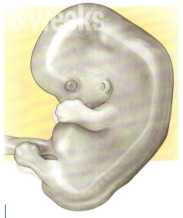

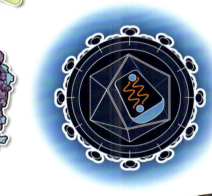

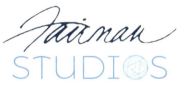

fairman
STUDIOS

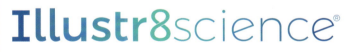

Illustr8science®

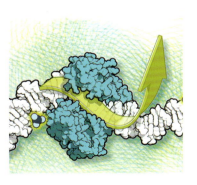

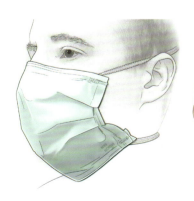

Engage.
Educate.
Communicate.

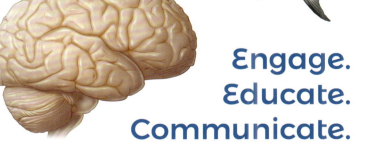

fairmanstudios.com · illustr8science.com · (781) 647-7510 · info@fairmanstudios.com · f ♥ in ⓘ @fairmanstudios

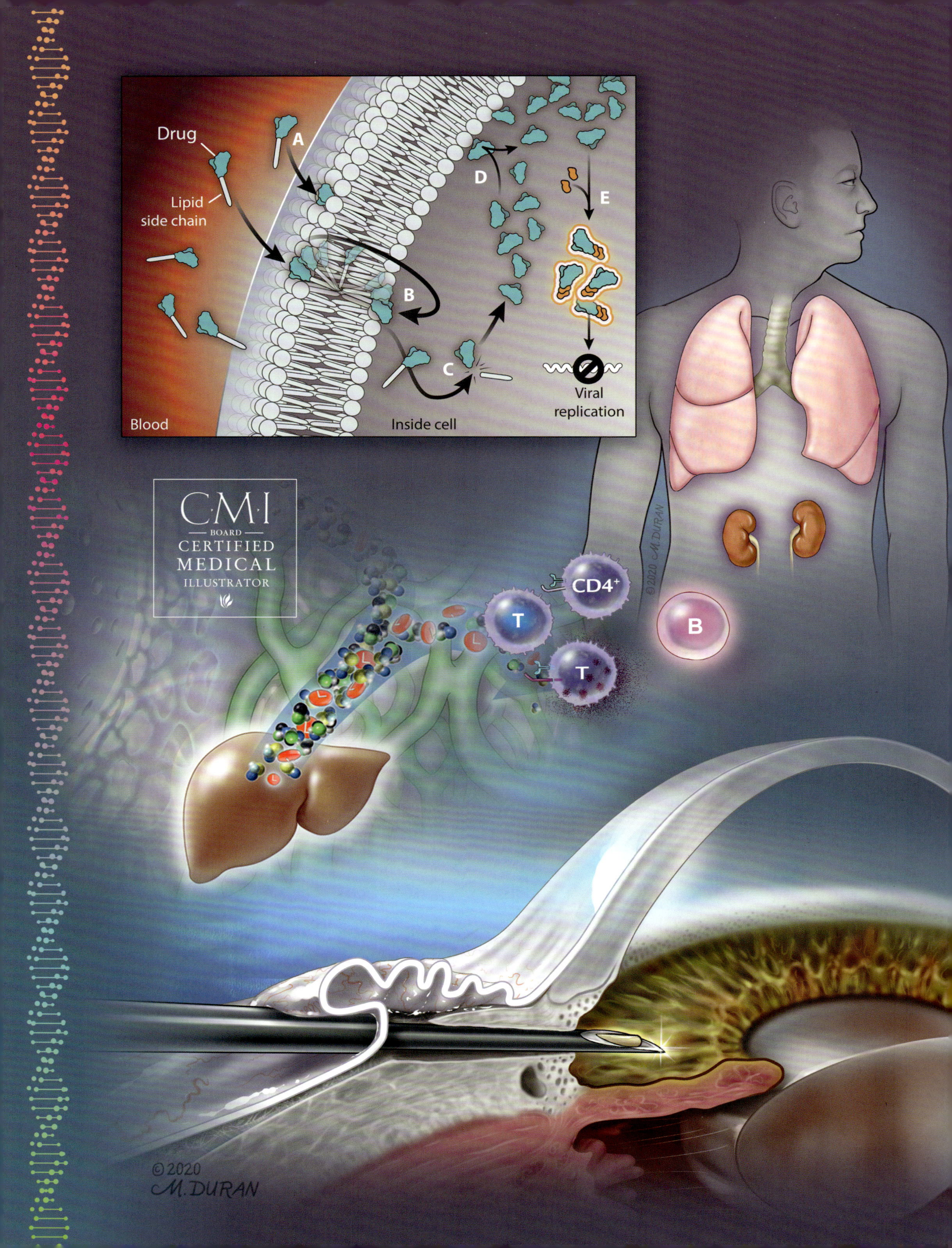

Drug

Lipid side chain

A

B

C

D

E

Viral replication

Blood

Inside cell

CD4+

T

T

B

CMI
BOARD
CERTIFIED
MEDICAL
ILLUSTRATOR

©2020

M. DURAN

©2020 M. DURAN

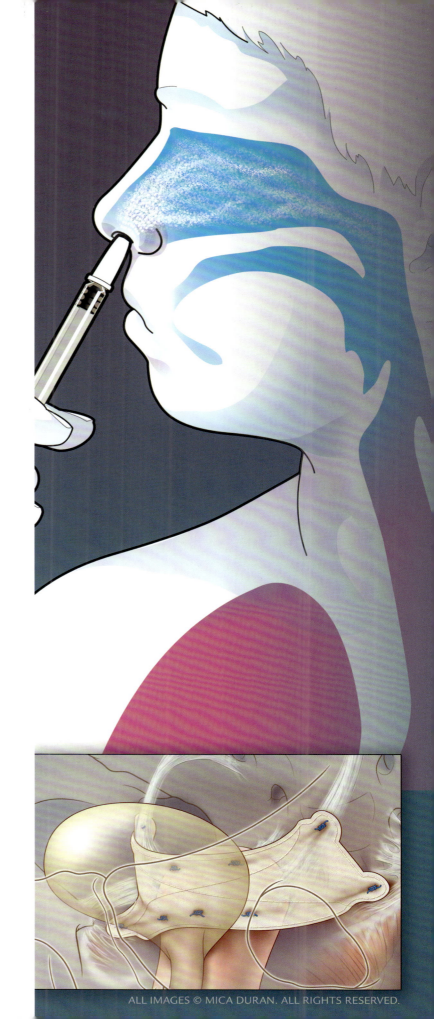

Let's work together

Representing the world's

medical and scientific experts

with hand-drawn illustration

for 20+ years.

PHARMACEUTICAL INDUSTRY

MEDICAL DEVICE SALES AND TRAINING

SCIENTIFIC PUBLICATIONS

MICA DURAN STUDIO

WWW.MICADURAN.COM

1-800-493-4553

ALL IMAGES © MICA DURAN. ALL RIGHTS RESERVED.

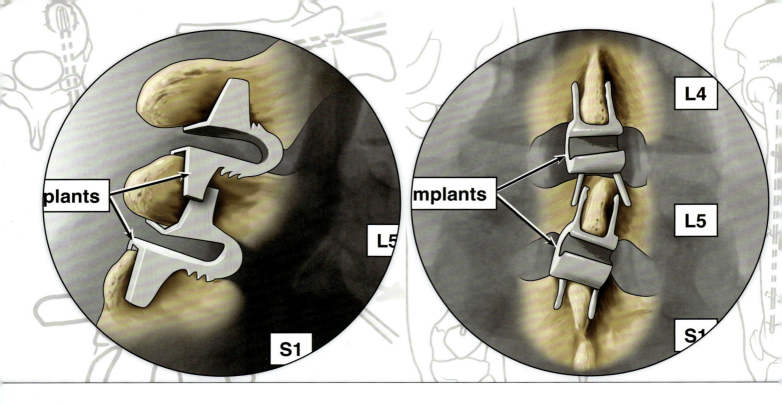

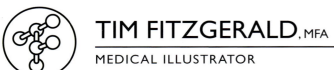

TIM FITZGERALD, MFA

MEDICAL ILLUSTRATOR

TIMFITZBIOART.COM
TIMFITZBIOART@GMAIL.COM
@TIMFITZ_BIOART
@TIMFITZ-BIOART

- EXHIBIT DESIGN -
- MEDICAL FILM COLORIZATION -
- SURGICAL ILLUSTRATION -
- STORYBOARD LAYOUT -

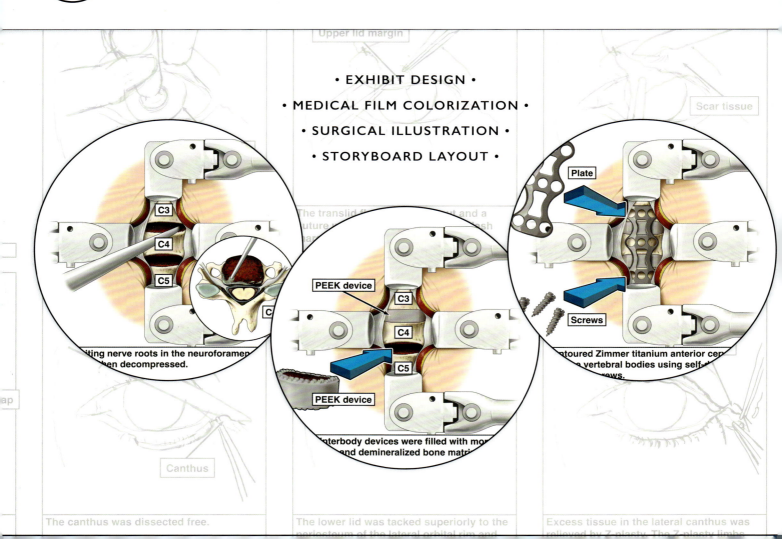

Medical device illustration & animation

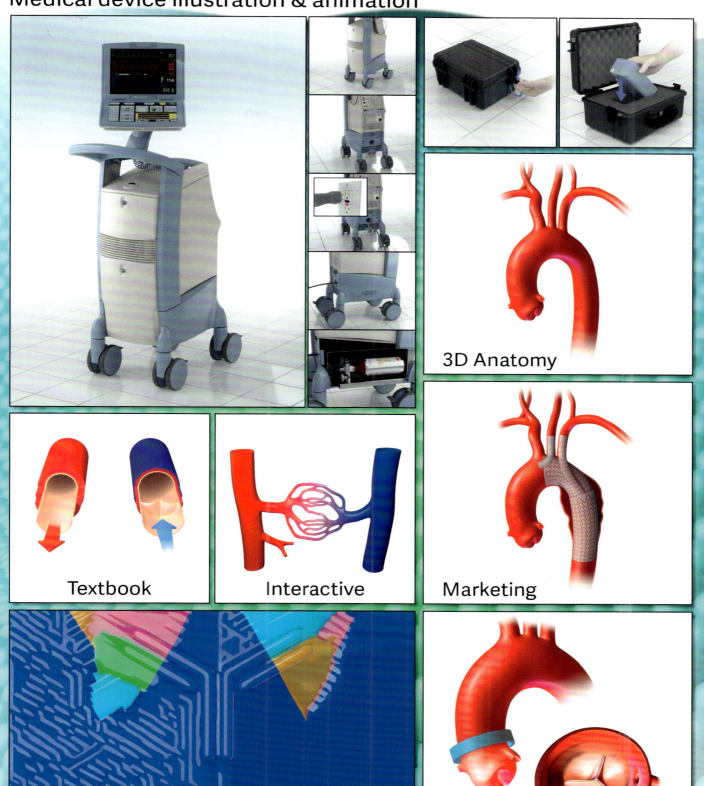

3D Anatomy

Textbook

Interactive

Marketing

Corporate fine art commissions

Education

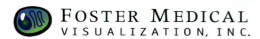

FOSTER MEDICAL
VISUALIZATION, INC.

USA - Stacey Endress
London - Juliette Lott

Represented by
illustrationx.com

1(646) 808-0205
+44 (0) 207-720-5202

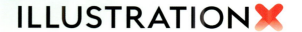

ILLUSTRATION X

stacey@illustrationx.com
juliette@illustrationx.com

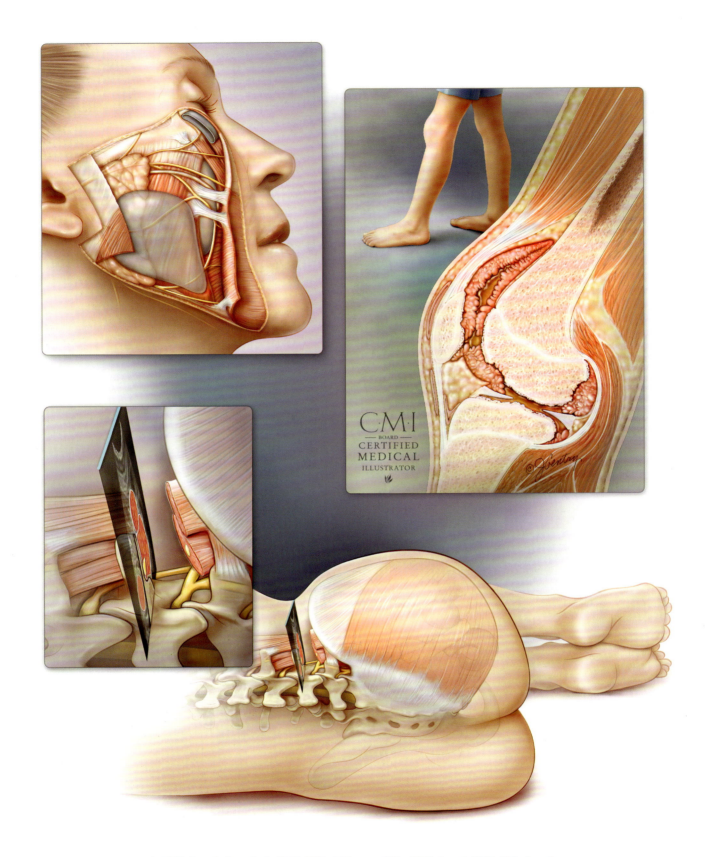

JENNIFER GENTRY

www.gentryvisualization.com

336.703.9343 | jennifer@gentryvisualization.com

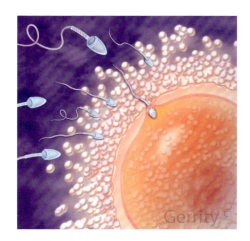
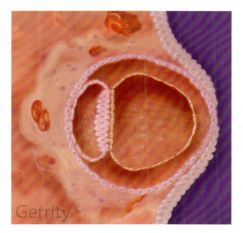
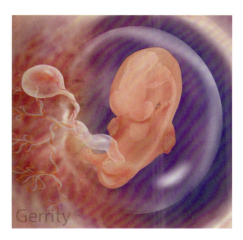
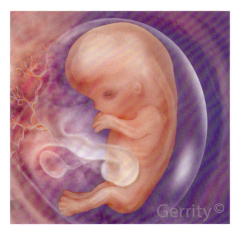
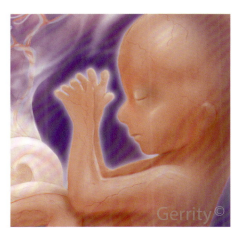
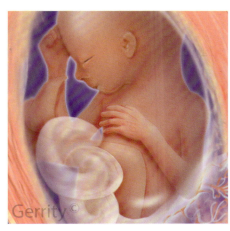
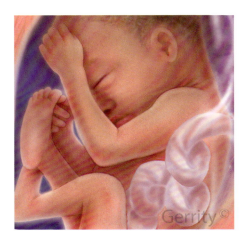
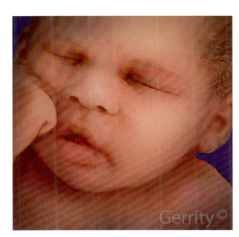
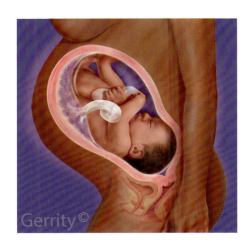

Gerrity | Connolly
CHICAGO
MEDICAL GRAPHICS
www.chicagomedicalgraphics.com | 281-304-0745

Peg Gerrity, MAMS, CMI
2D Medical Illustration
2D Animation
peg@peggerrity.com

Melanie Connolly, MS
3D Medical Illustration
3D Animation
melanie@mecovisuals.com

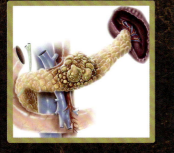
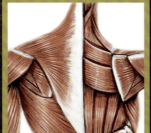
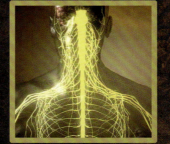
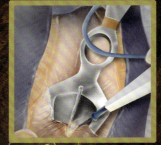

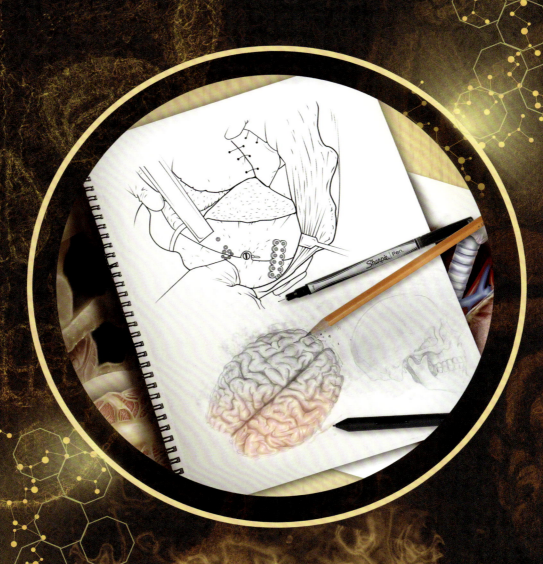

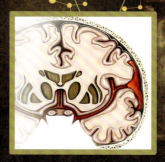

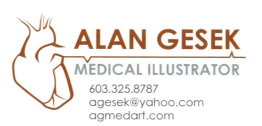

ALAN GESEK
MEDICAL ILLUSTRATOR

603.325.8787
agesek@yahoo.com
agmedart.com

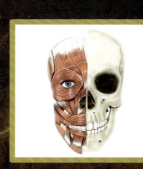

CM·I
BOARD
CERTIFIED
MEDICAL
ILLUSTRATOR

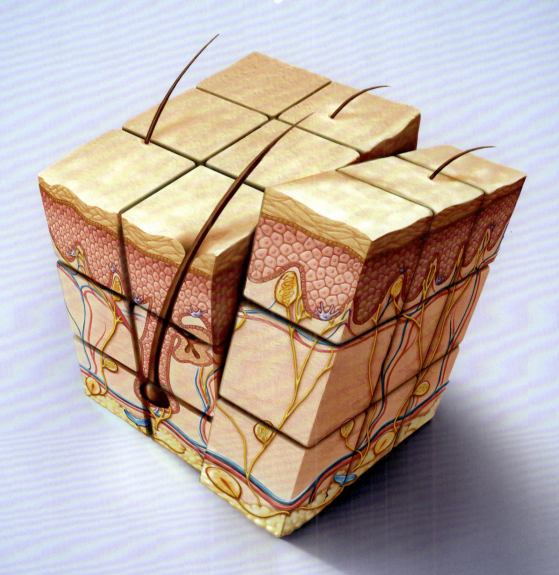

**YOUR STORY SHOULD BE
EASIER TO UNDERSTAND**

GOTTLIEBVISUALS.COM

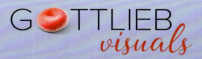

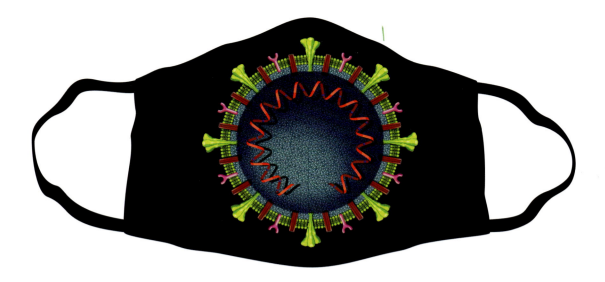

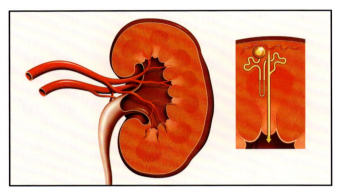

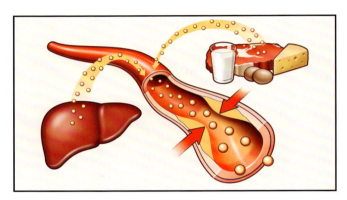

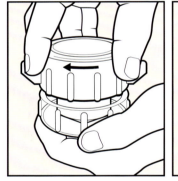

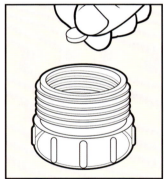

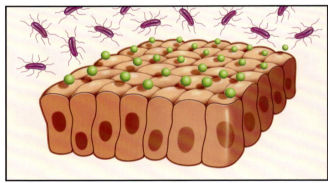

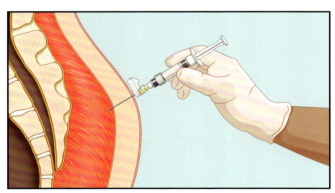

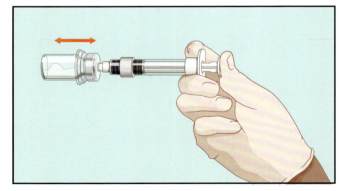

Winner of the 2020 Rx Award of Excellence for *Educational Animation* and for *Physician Education*

- MOTION GRAPHICS
- EXPLAINERS
- INFOGRAPHICS

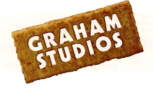

WILLIAM GRAHAM
818-398-4747
www.grahamstudios.net

Chris Gralapp MA, CMI

eyeart@chrisgralapp.com
www.chrisgralapp.com

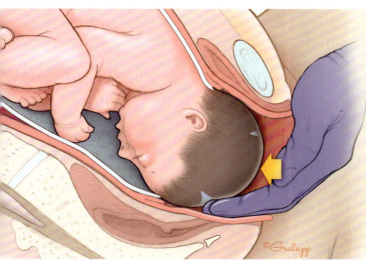

I 've been privileged to work with Chris for over 15 years. She has provided key medical illustrations for a wide variety of medical negligence cases. Chris' illustrations are meticulously medically accurate but are also easily understandable by the jury. Chris is easy to work with and can adapt our experts' thinking into graphic reality. I greatly value Chris' input on our team.

Elizabeth A. Leedom
Attorney / Director
Bennett Bigelow & Leedom P.S.
Seattle

I have worked with Chris for over ten years, and she is a true professional. Her art is amazing and recognized the world over. Her work in our book received a reviewer score of 99 out of 100, 5 Stars.

Timothy Y. Hiscock
Executive Editor
Thieme Publishers
New York, NY

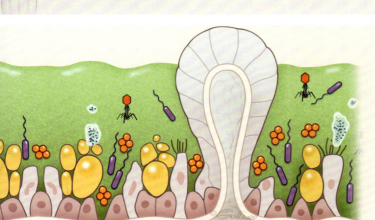

Chris's illustrations have added great impact to my primary research papers, review articles and book chapters. She quickly and expertly converts scientific and medical concepts into beautifully clear images. Chris communicates very well, is highly responsive, and respects timeline pressures. She is a real pleasure to work with.

John Fahy, MD
Professor and Director, UCSF Airway Clinical Research Center

Chris continues to impress. She is extremely easy to work with, and the utmost professional. Her anatomy knowledge is excellent, and she has an exceptional aptitude for understanding and illustrating complex anatomy. Her illustrations add great value. We love working with Chris, and would highly recommend her to anyone looking for medical illustration services.

Eric Savitsky, MD
UCLA Professor Emergency Medicine/Pediatric Emergency Medicine

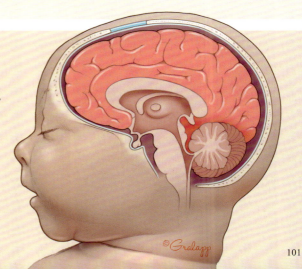

MICHELE GRAHAM

www.michelegraham.com   (970) 775-3557   michele@internalcolors.com

CMI
— BOARD —
CERTIFIED
MEDICAL
ILLUSTRATOR

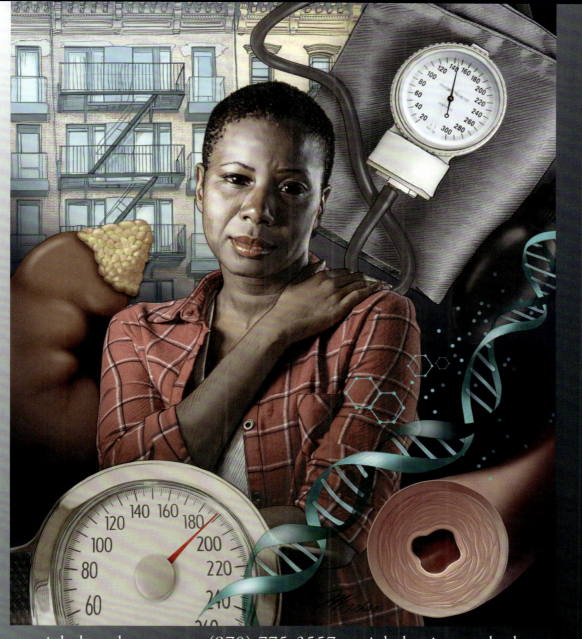

www.michelegraham.com   (970) 775-3557   michele@internalcolors.com

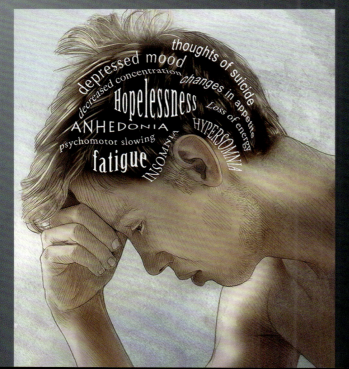

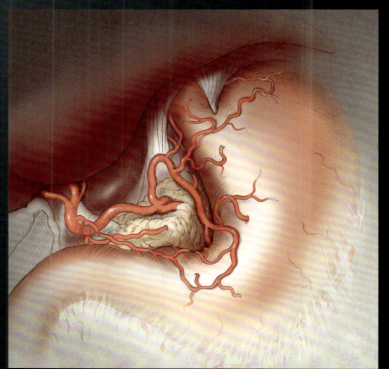

Concept development, storyboards, award winning medical and biological illustration for advertising, editorial, patient education and textbooks

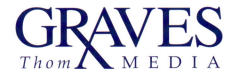

Thom Graves
917.912.4894
thom@thomgravescreative.com
www.thomgravescreative.com

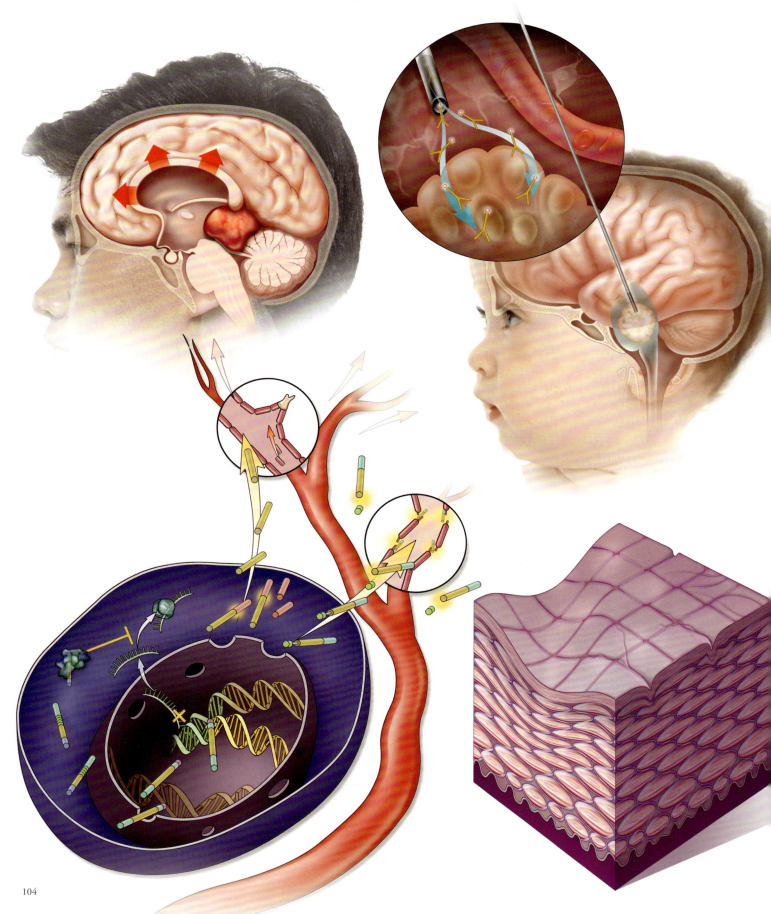

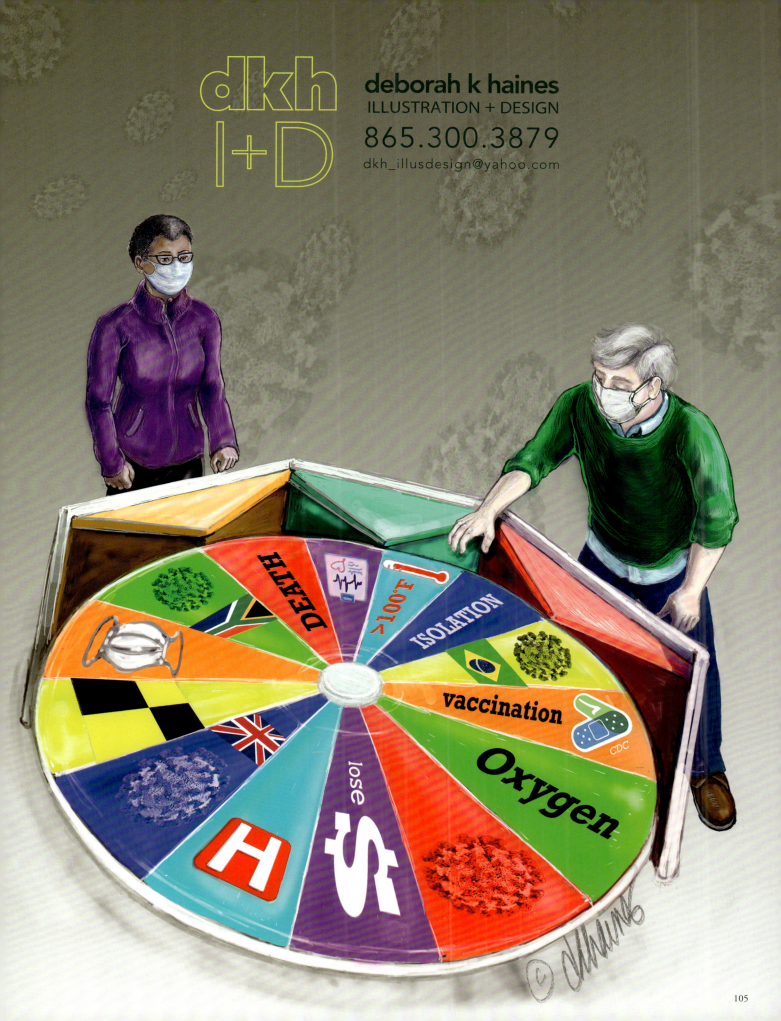

dkh
I+D

deborah k haines
ILLUSTRATION + DESIGN
865.300.3879
dkh_illusdesign@yahoo.com

105

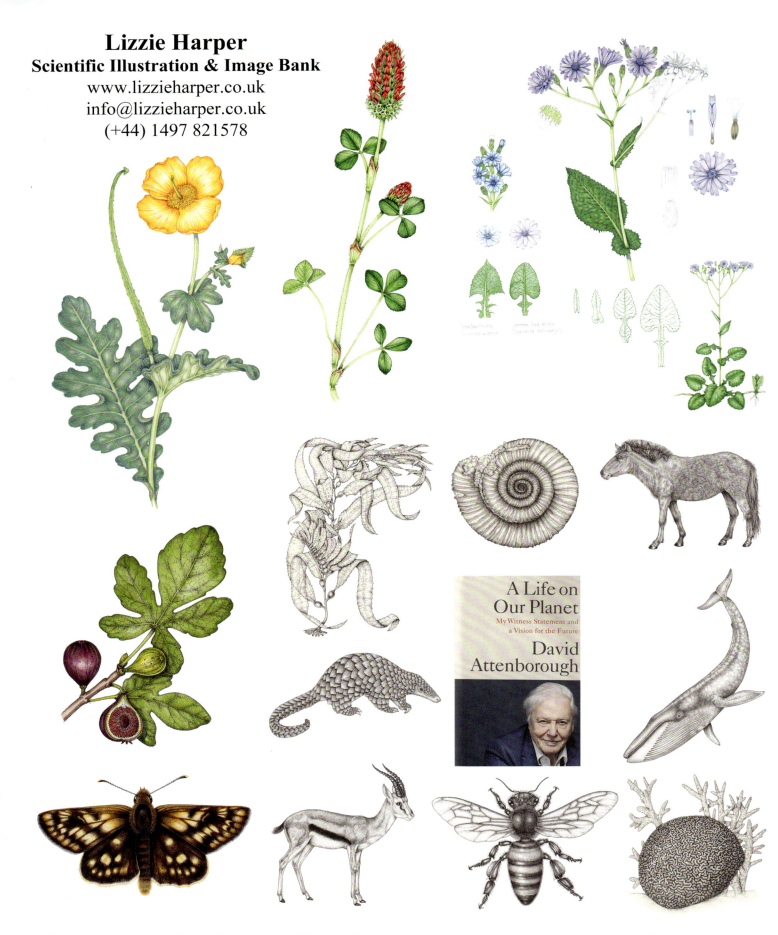

Lizzie Harper
Scientific Illustration & Image Bank

www.lizzieharper.co.uk
info@lizzieharper.co.uk
(+44) 1497 821578

A Life on
Our Planet
My Witness Statement and
a Vision for the Future

David
Attenborough

Lizzie Harper is a traditional Botanical and Natural Science Illustrator working in watercolor, pen and ink, and graphite. She has an online image bank of over 1500 illustrations available for licensed re-use at www.lizzieharper.co.uk/galleries/ Please email her with your illustration needs & project ideas.

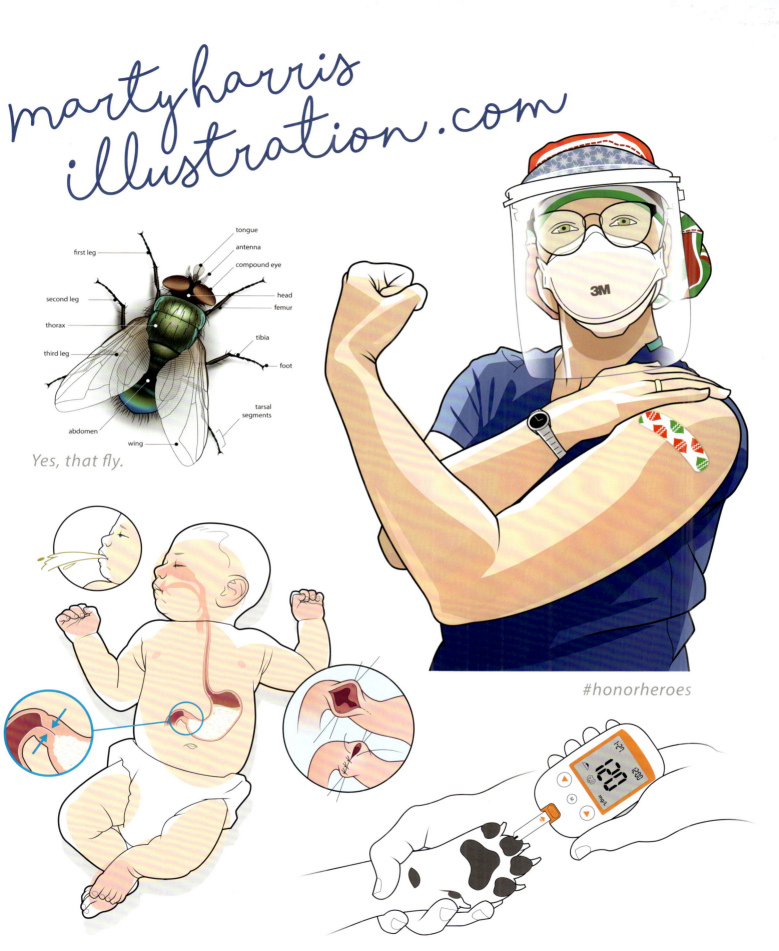

martyharris
illustration.com

tongue
first leg
antenna
compound eye
head
second leg
femur
thorax
tibia
third leg
foot
abdomen
wing
tarsal segments

Yes, that fly.

#honorheroes

martyharrisillustration@gmail.com   +1 952-221-5212

BRIAN HARROLD

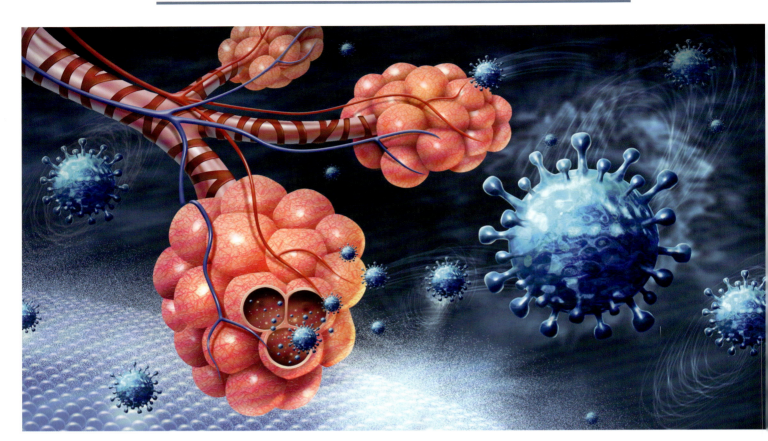

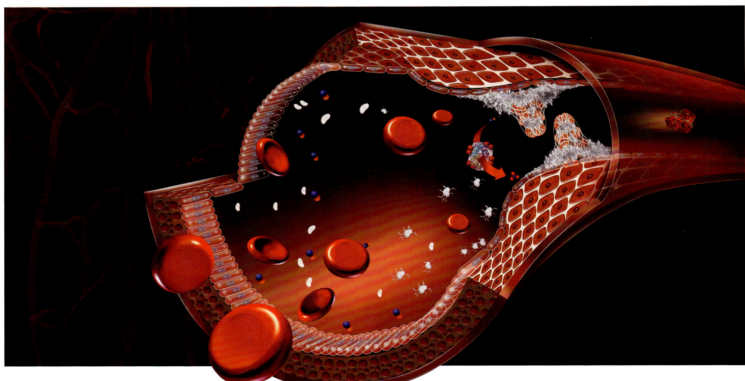

brianharrold.com · berugraphics.com · berugraphics@gmail.com · 917.375.2086

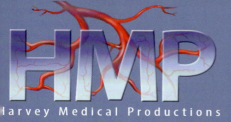

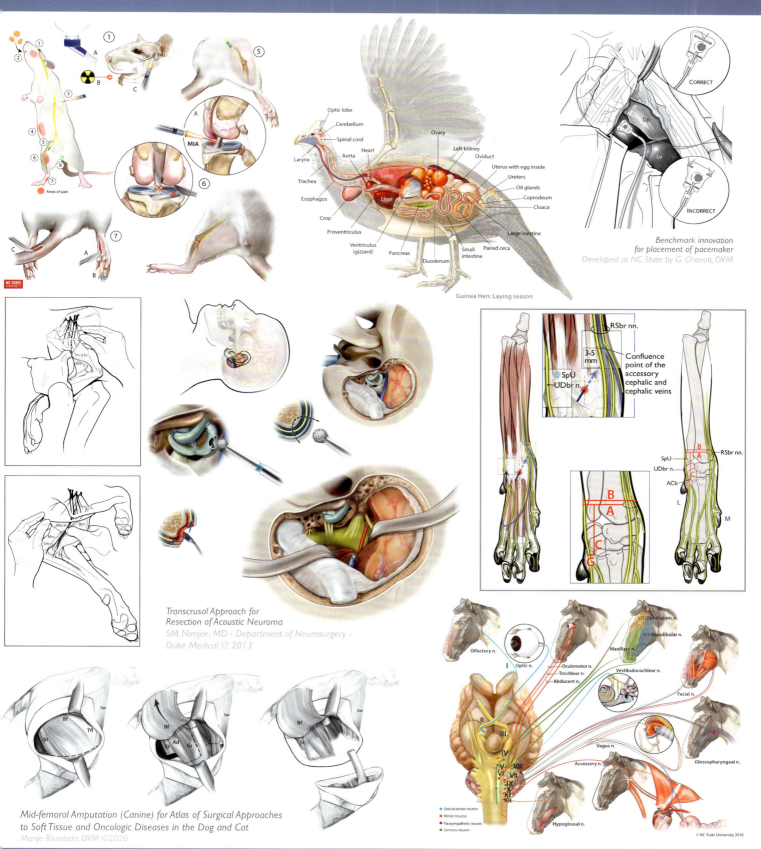

Benchmark innovation
for placement of pacemaker
Developed at NC State by G. Chanoit, DVM

Guinea Hen: Laying season

Optic lobe
Cerebellum
Spinal cord
Larynx
Aorta
Heart
Trachea
Esophagus
Lung
Liver
Crop
Proventriculus
Ventriculus
(gizzard)
Pancreas
Duodenum
Small
intestine
Ovary
Left kidney
Oviduct
Uterus with egg inside
Ureters
Oil glands
Coprodeum
Cloaca
Large intestine
Paired ceca

CORRECT
INCORRECT

Areas of pain

Transcrusal Approach for
Resection of Acoustic Neuroma
*SM Nimjee, MD - Department of Neurosurgery -
Duke Medical © 2013*

RSbr nn.
3-5
mm
Confluence
point of the
accessory
cephalic and
cephalic veins
SpU
UDbr n.

Mid-femoral Amputation (Canine) for Atlas of Surgical Approaches
to Soft Tissue and Oncologic Diseases in the Dog and Cat
Marije Risselada, DVM ©2020

Olfactory n.
Optic n.
Oculomotor n.
Trochlear n.
Abducent n.
VII) Ophthalmic n.
VIII) Mandibular n.
Maxillary n.
Vestibulocochlear n.
Facial n.
Vagus n.
Accessory n.
Glossopharyngeal n.
Hypoglossal n.

Special senses neuron
Motor neuron
Parasympathetic neuron
Sensory neuron

© NC State University 2016

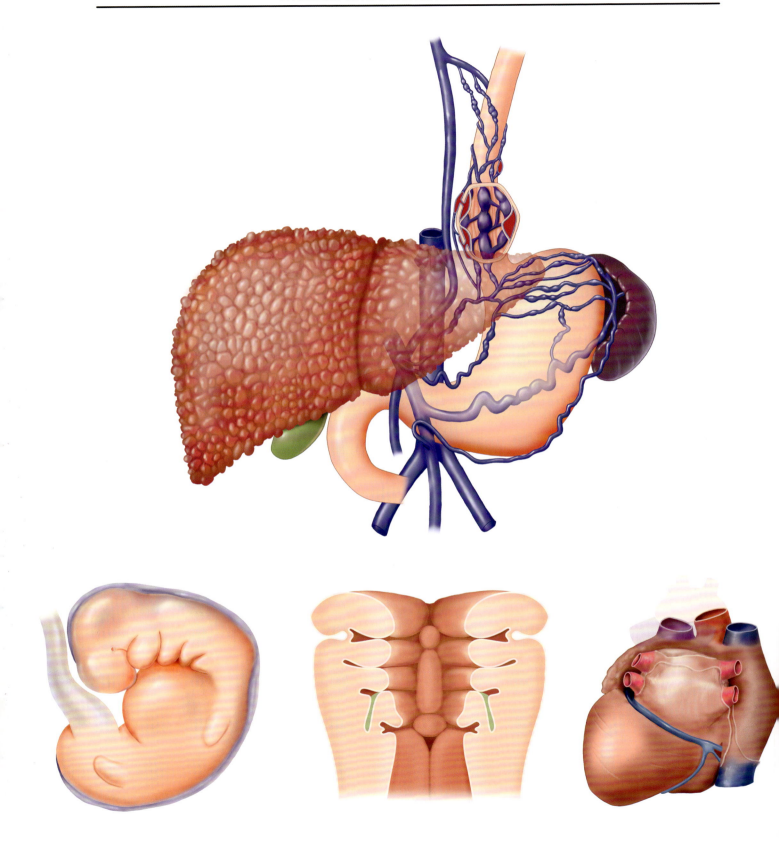

www.suzanne-hayes.com   303-681-8828   suzannehayes01@gmail.com

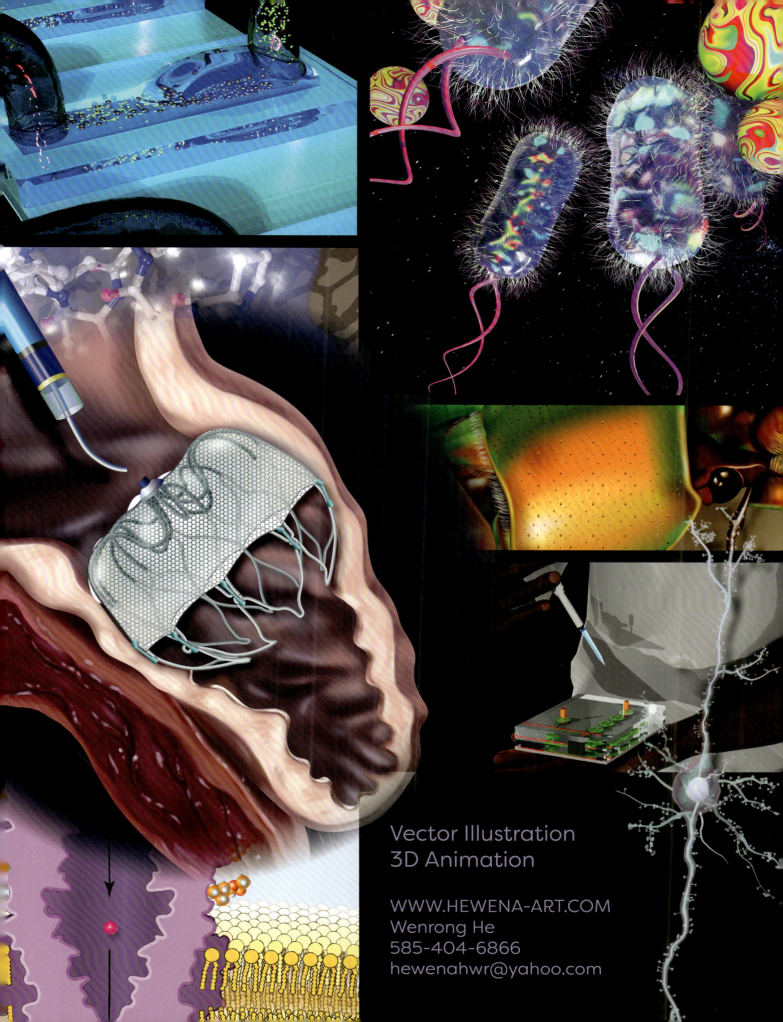

Vector Illustration
3D Animation

WWW.HEWENA-ART.COM
Wenrong He
585-404-6866
hewenahwr@yahoo.com

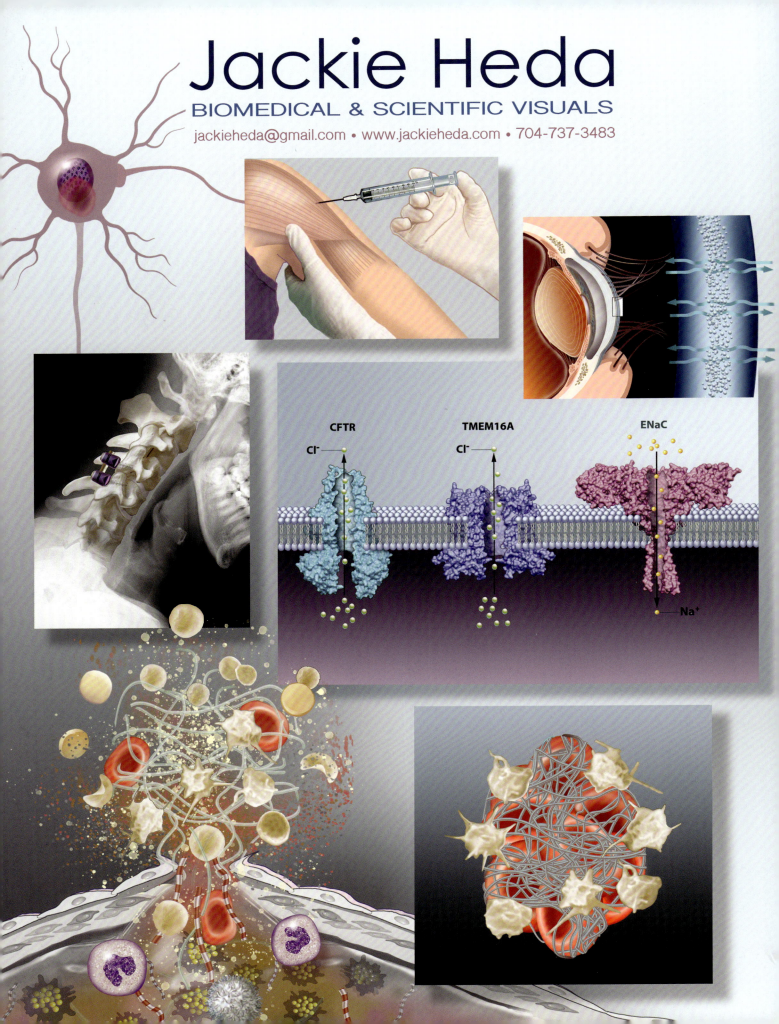

Jackie Heda
BIOMEDICAL & SCIENTIFIC VISUALS
jackieheda@gmail.com • www.jackieheda.com • 704-737-3483

CFTR

TMEM16A

ENaC

Cl⁻

Cl⁻

Na⁺

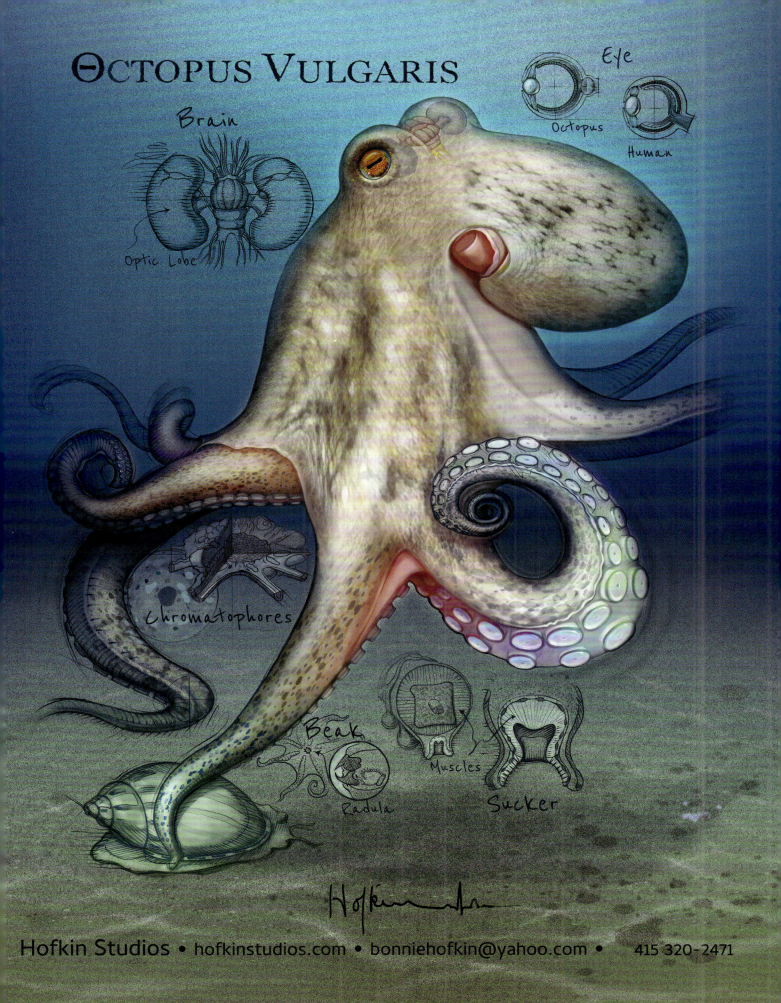

ΘCTOPUS VULGARIS

Brain

Optic Lobe

Eye

Octopus

Human

Chromatophores

Beak

Radula

Muscles

Sucker

Hofkin Studios • hofkinstudios.com • bonniehofkin@yahoo.com •   415 320-2471

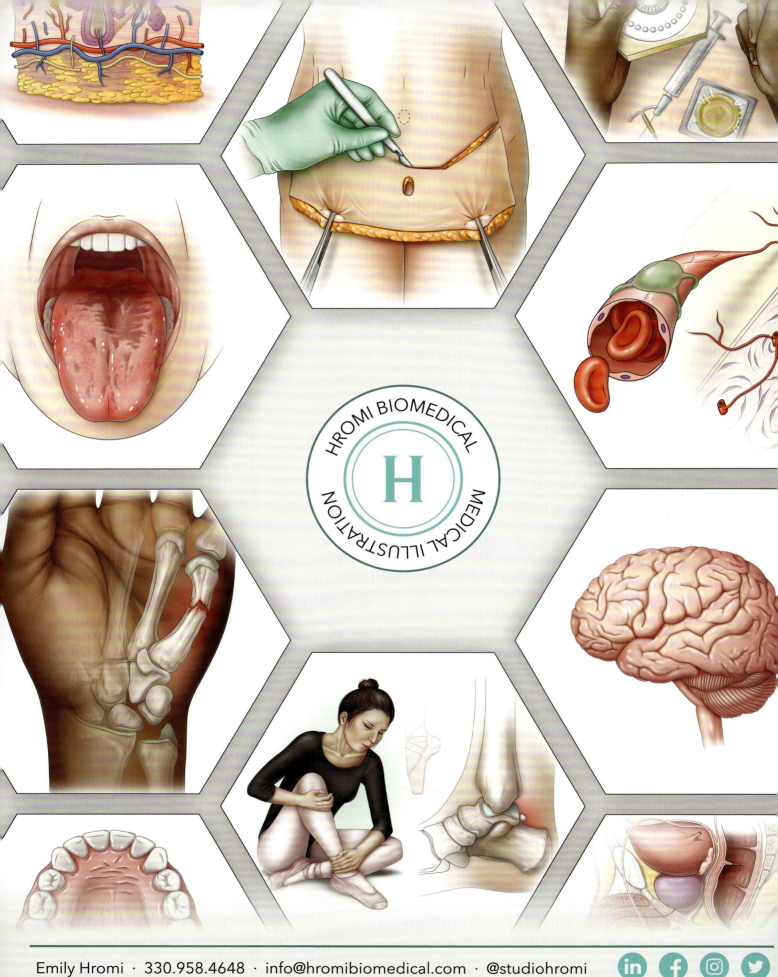

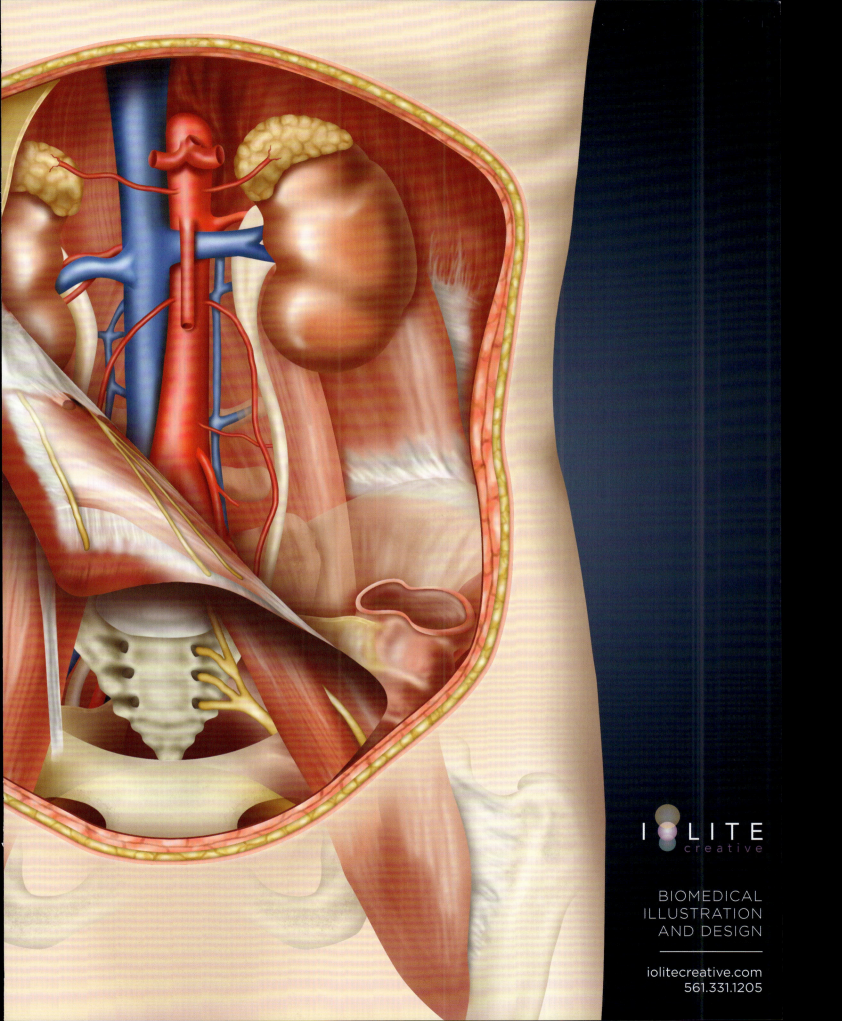

I LITE
creative

BIOMEDICAL
ILLUSTRATION
AND DESIGN

iolitecreative.com
561.331.1205

nícole jones
medical art & design

111jones@verizon.net
www.NicoleJonesArt.com
610-213-8550

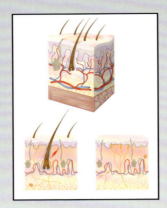

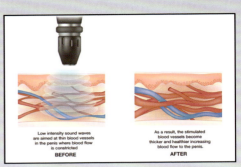

Low intensity sound waves are aimed at thin blood vessels in the penis where blood flow is constricted
BEFORE

As a result, the stimulated blood vessels become thicker and healthier increasing blood flow to the penis.
AFTER

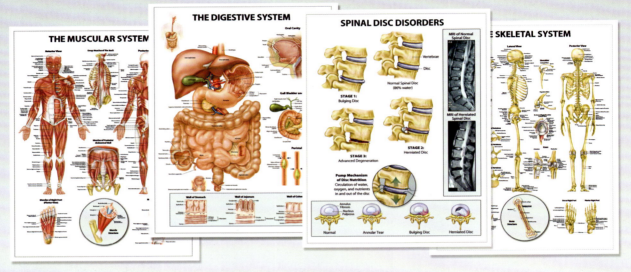

THE MUSCULAR SYSTEM

THE DIGESTIVE SYSTEM

SPINAL DISC DISORDERS

THE SKELETAL SYSTEM

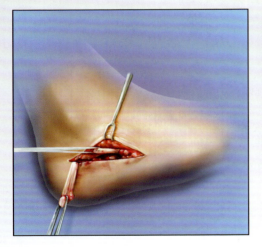

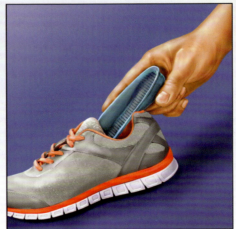

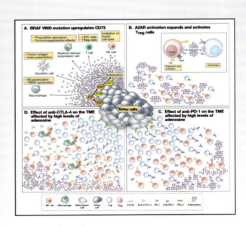

NICOLE M JONES
Medical & Scientific Illustrator

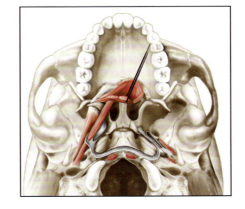

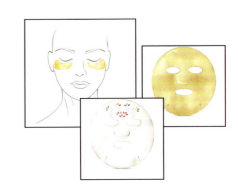

116

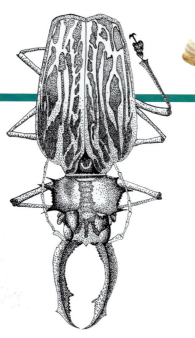

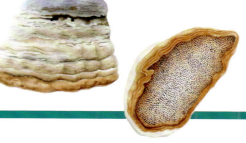

JOAN'S LIFE ART

www.joanslifeart.info

(603) 523-9274
thomsonj793@gmail.com

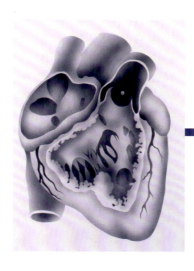

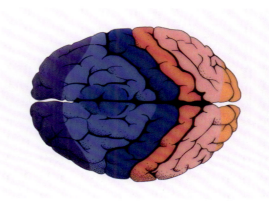

FUNGI
BOTANICALS
FIELD GUIDES
PATIENT EDUCATION
MEDICAL

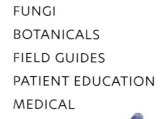

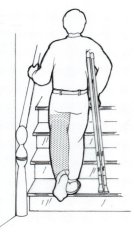

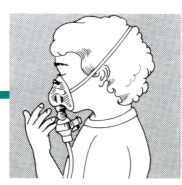

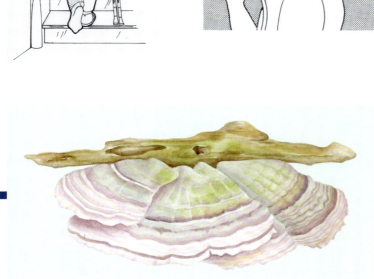

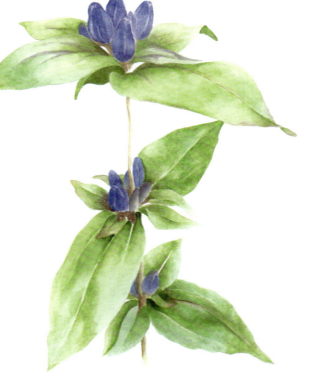

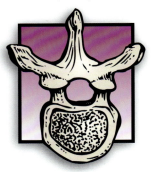

WENDY BETH JACKELOW
MFA, CMI, FAMI

Medical & Scientific Illustration

(718) 273-0002
wendy@wbjackelowstudios.com
www.wbjackelowstudios.com

CMI
— BOARD —
CERTIFIED
MEDICAL
ILLUSTRATOR

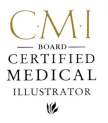

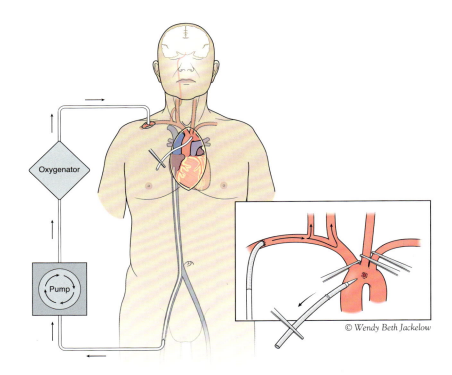

© Wendy Beth Jackelow

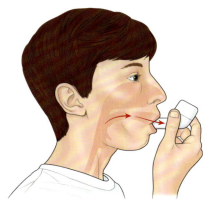

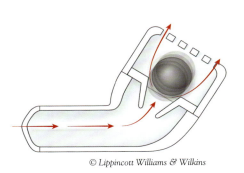

© Lippincott Williams & Wilkins

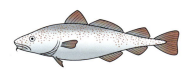

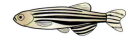

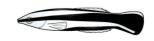

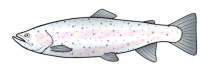

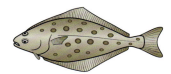

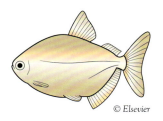

© Elsevier

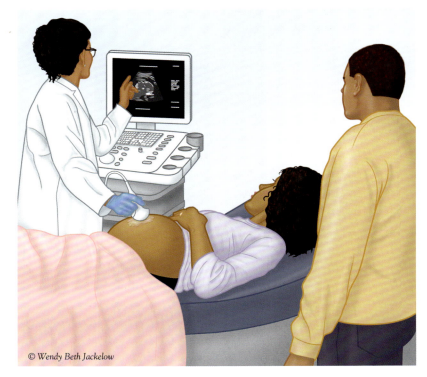

© Wendy Beth Jackelow

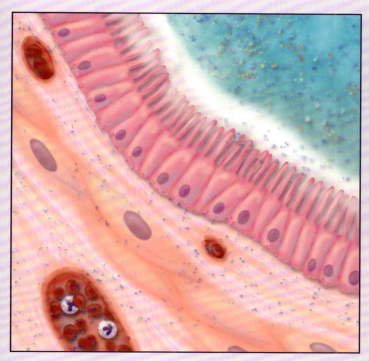
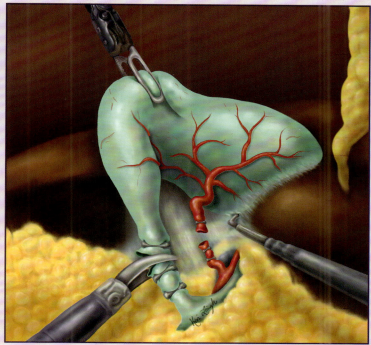
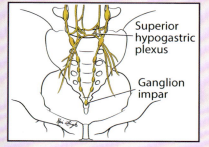

Superior hypogastric plexus

Ganglion impar

Keri *KL* Leigh
Biomedical Creations

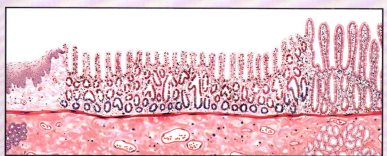

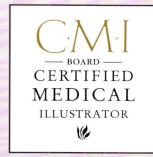

C·M·I
— BOARD —
CERTIFIED
MEDICAL
ILLUSTRATOR

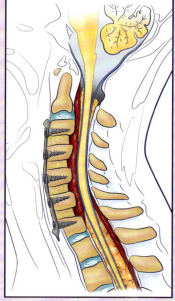

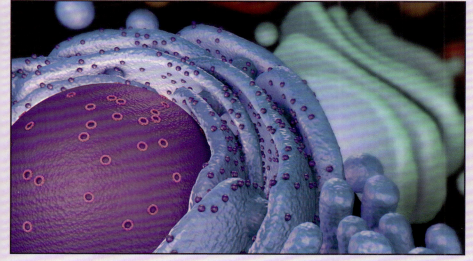

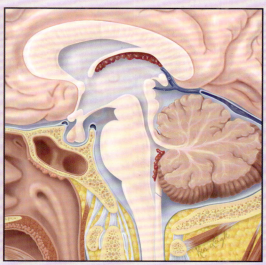

www.klbiomedcreations.com   Keri Leigh Jones, MSMI, CMI   kerileigh@klbiomedcreations.com

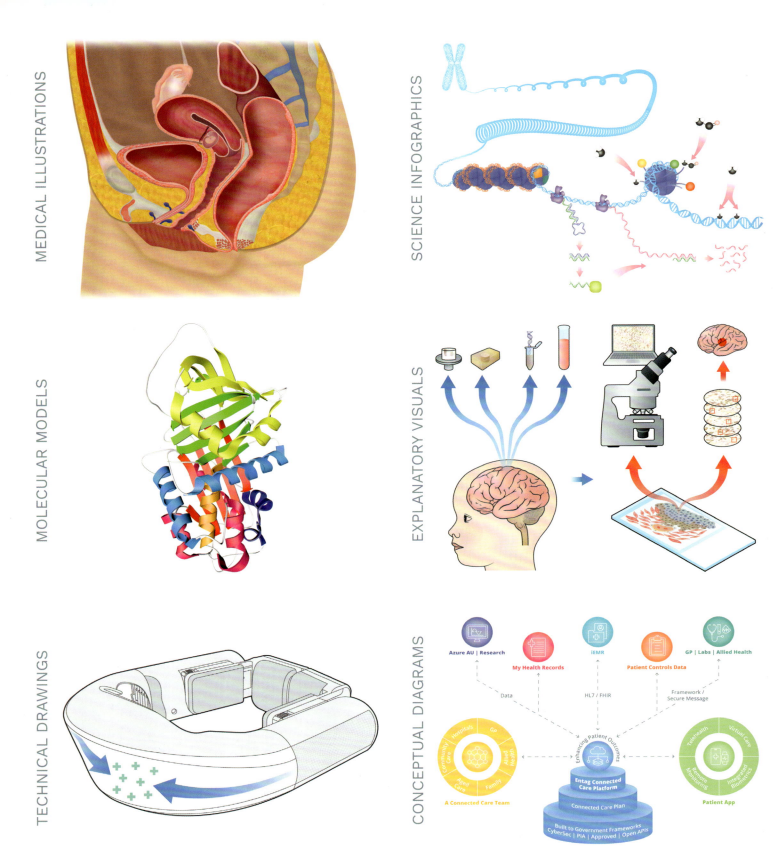

MEDICAL ILLUSTRATIONS

SCIENCE INFOGRAPHICS

MOLECULAR MODELS

EXPLANATORY VISUALS

TECHNICAL DRAWINGS

CONCEPTUAL DIAGRAMS

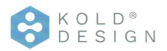

KOLD® DESIGN

PROVIDING CUSTOM-MADE VISUAL STORIES IN SCIENCE, EDUCATION, TECHNOLOGY, AND HEALTHCARE

www.kold.design • +44 (0)75 6142 7092 • info@kold.design

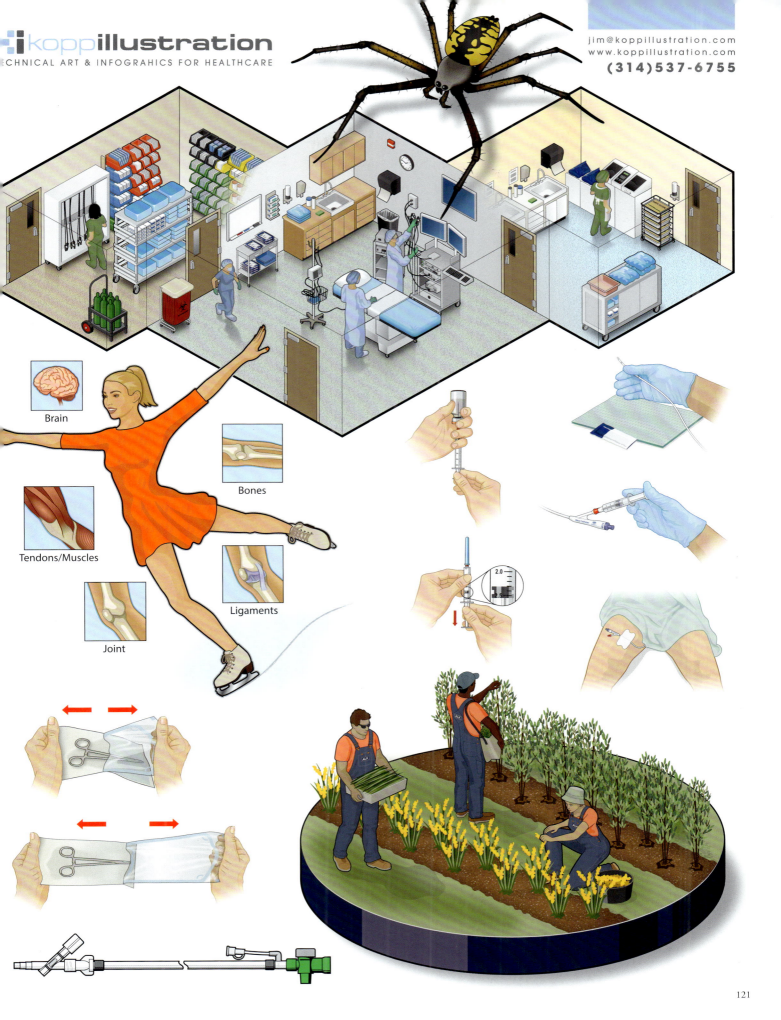

koppillustration
TECHNICAL ART & INFOGRAHICS FOR HEALTHCARE

jim@koppillustration.com
www.koppillustration.com
(314)537-6755

Brain

Bones

Tendons/Muscles

Ligaments

Joint

2.0

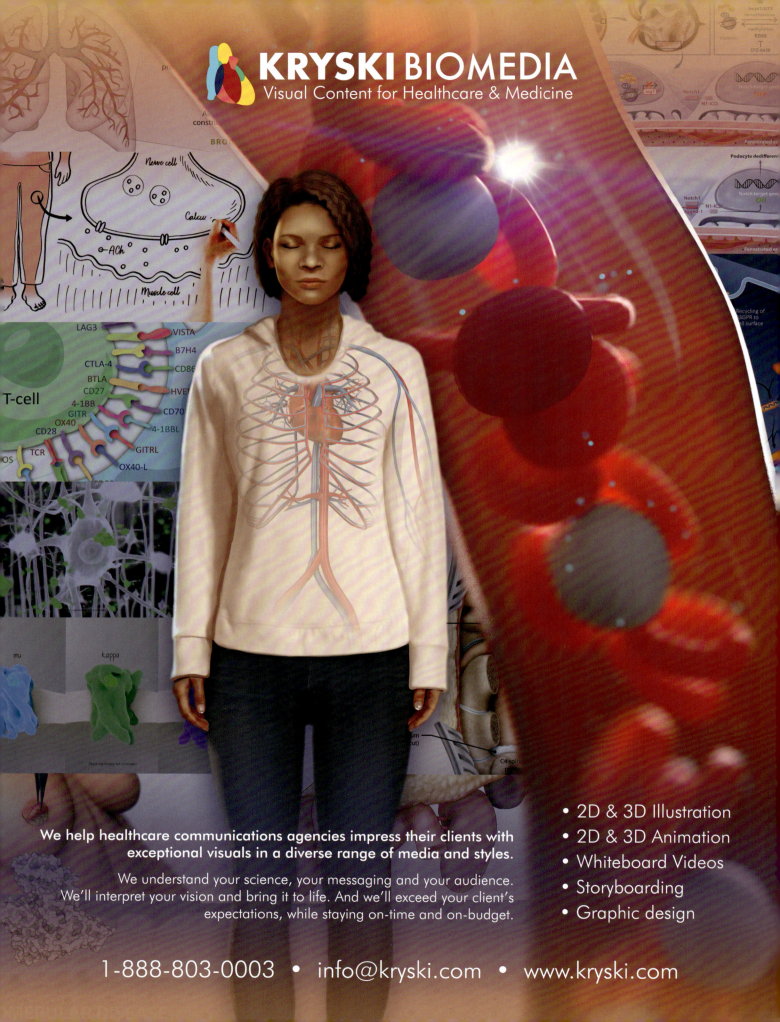

KRYSKI BIOMEDIA
Visual Content for Healthcare & Medicine

We help healthcare communications agencies impress their clients with exceptional visuals in a diverse range of media and styles.

We understand your science, your messaging and your audience. We'll interpret your vision and bring it to life. And we'll exceed your client's expectations, while staying on-time and on-budget.

- 2D & 3D Illustration
- 2D & 3D Animation
- Whiteboard Videos
- Storyboarding
- Graphic design

1-888-803-0003 • info@kryski.com • www.kryski.com

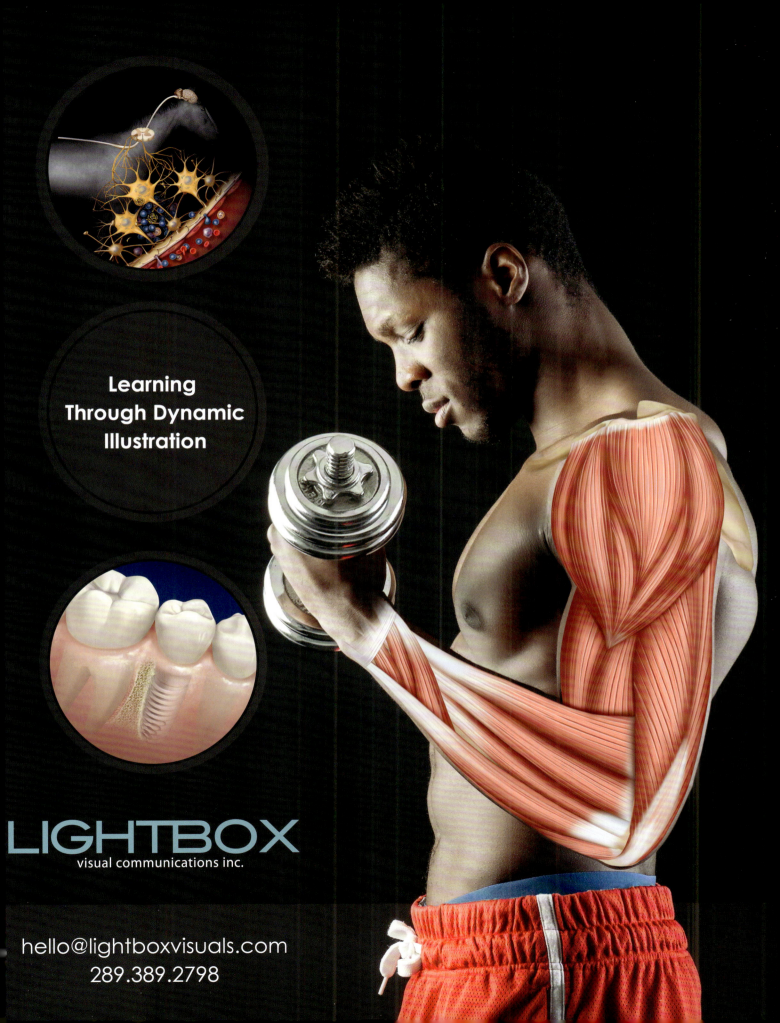

Learning
Through Dynamic
Illustration

LIGHTBOX
visual communications inc.

hello@lightboxvisuals.com
289.389.2798

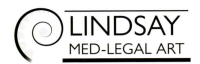

Begin your no obligation case review at
LindsayMedArt.com

We turn medical records into compelling visuals.

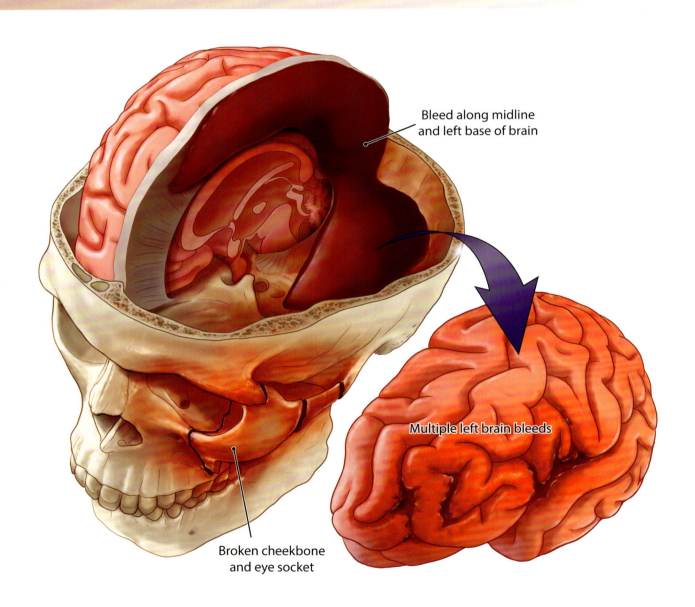

Bleed along midline and left base of brain

Multiple left brain bleeds

Broken cheekbone and eye socket

Custom images for catastrophic injury, wrongful death, and medical malpractice cases.
Contact@LindsayMedArt.com   308-293-6828

124

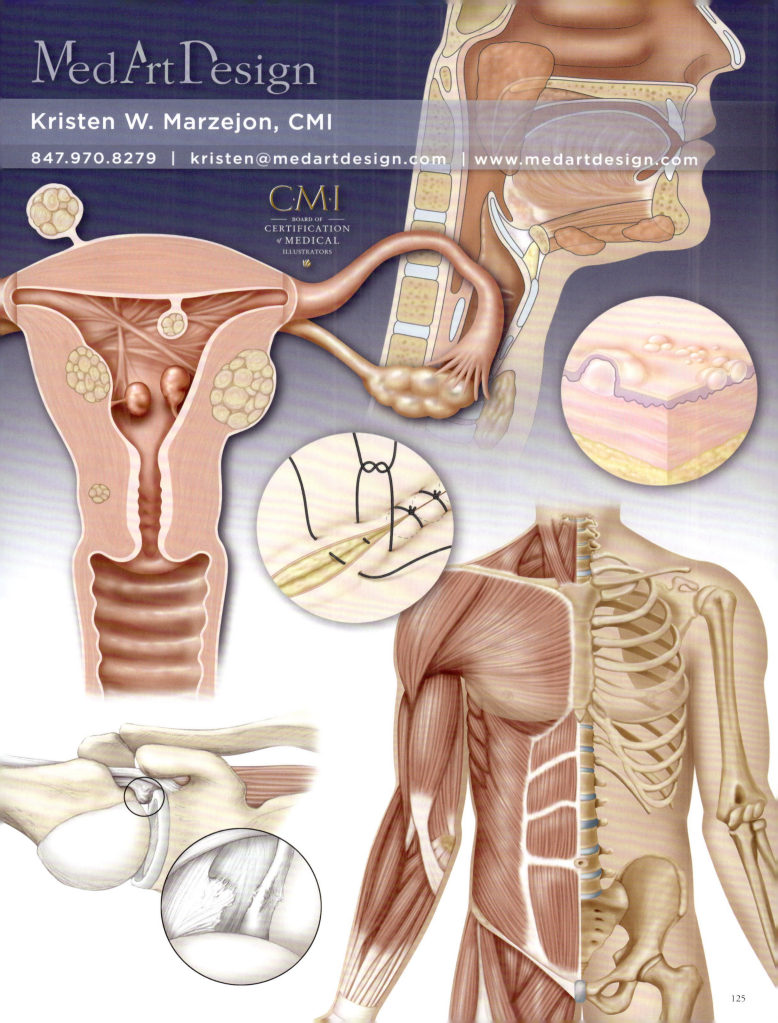

MedArtDesign

Kristen W. Marzejon, CMI

847.970.8279 | kristen@medartdesign.com | www.medartdesign.com

CMI
BOARD OF
CERTIFICATION
of MEDICAL
ILLUSTRATORS

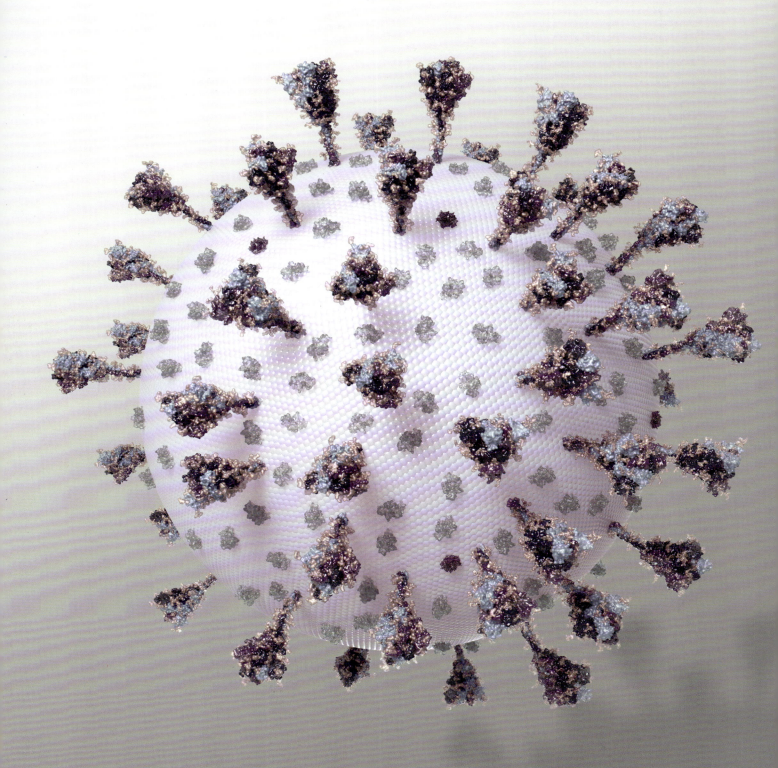

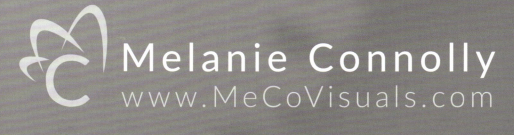

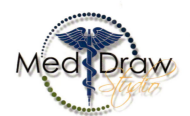
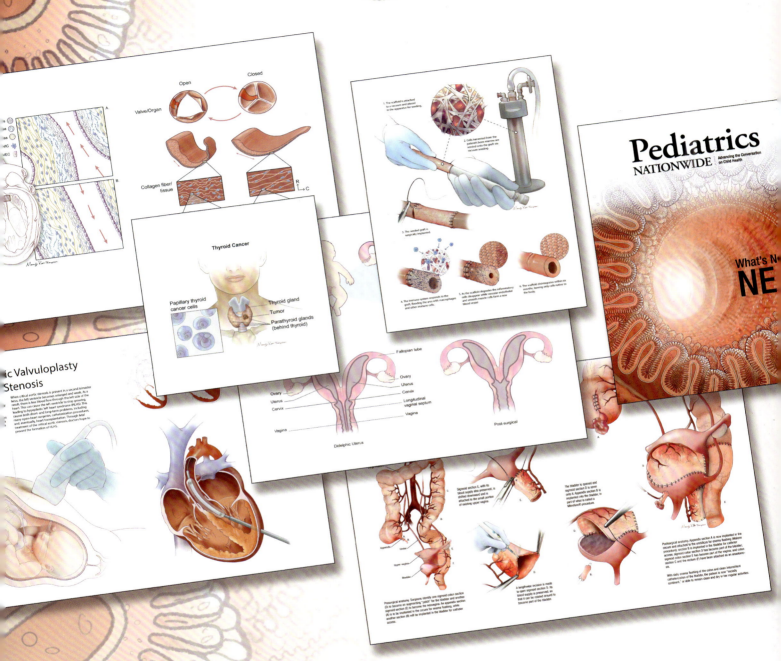

Simplifying Science

""Myself and co-authors are very impressed with your final drawing of the PDA closure device, and we thank you for your work on this. The manuscript has been accepted for publication in the Journal of Pediatrics. I truly think your drawing was a major selling point and one of the reasons for the acceptance – so thank you!"

Dr. Carl H Backes, M.D.
Departments of Cardiology and Neonatology
Nationwide Children's Hospital - The Ohio State University Wexner Medical Center

©2021 Mandy Root-Thompson/MedDraw Studio

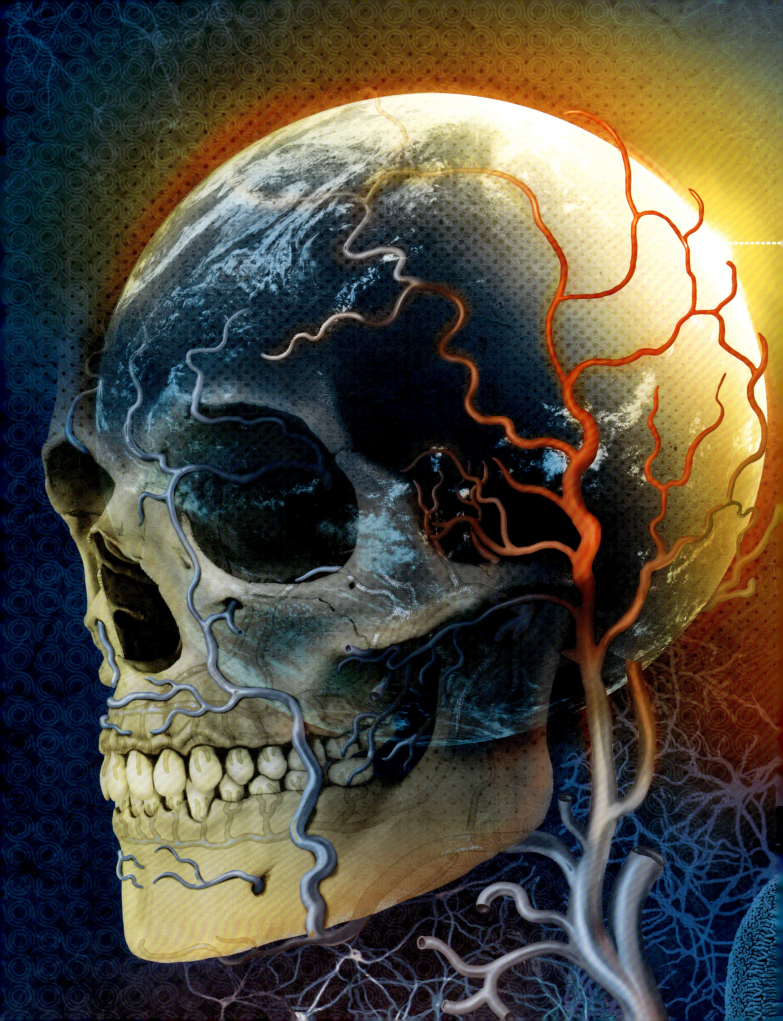

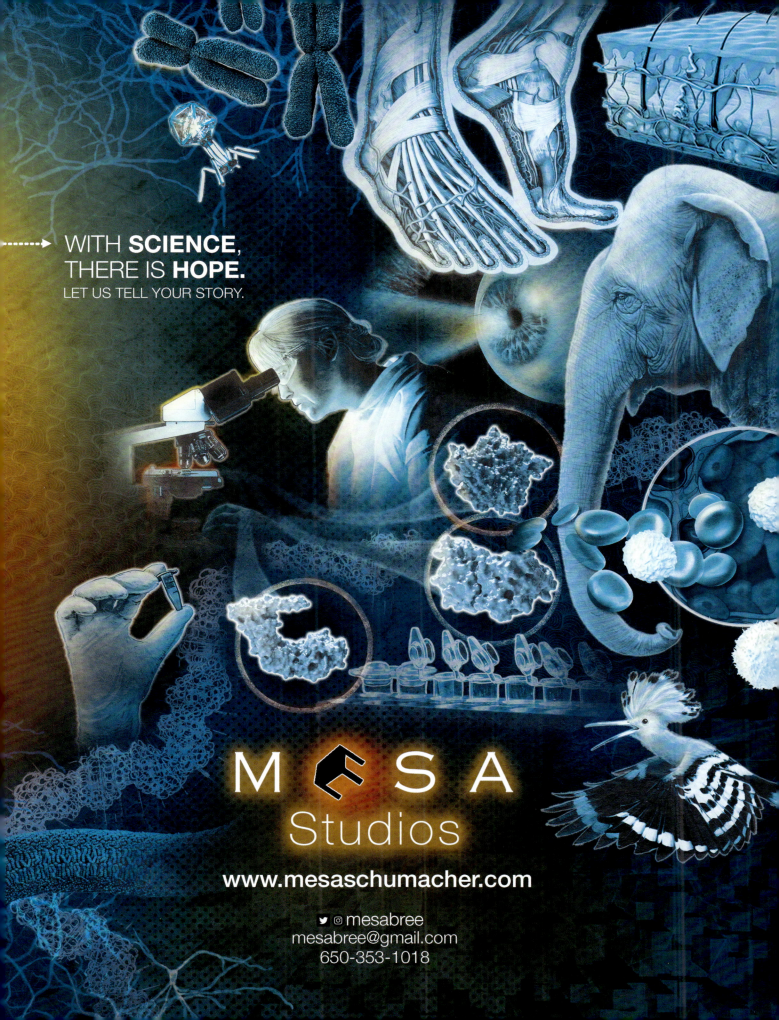

Fran Milner
Medical Illustration & Design
www.franimation.com • fran_milner@me.com • (470) 258-0340

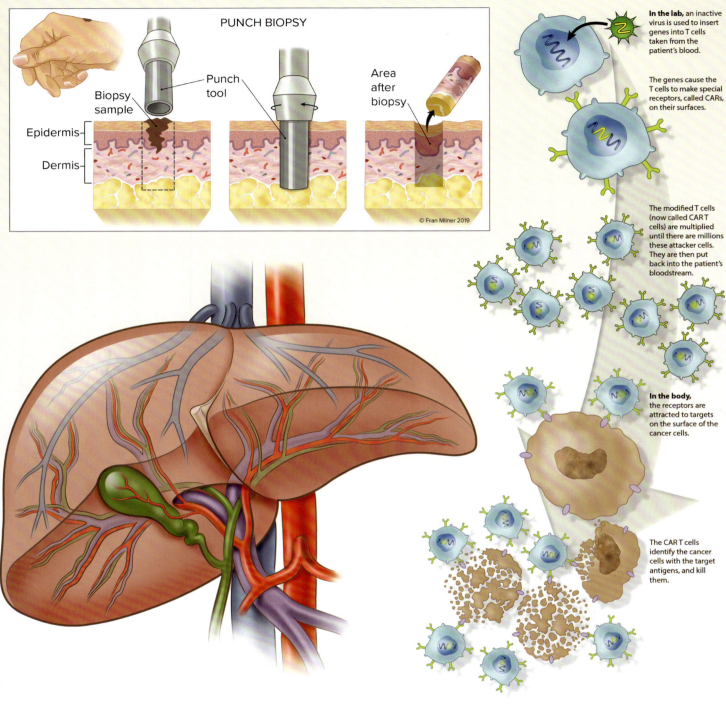

PUNCH BIOPSY

Biopsy sample

Punch tool

Epidermis

Dermis

Area after biopsy

© Fran Milner 2019

In the lab, an inactive virus is used to insert genes into T cells taken from the patient's blood.

The genes cause the T cells to make special receptors, called CARs, on their surfaces.

The modified T cells (now called CAR T cells) are multiplied until there are millions these attacker cells. They are then put back into the patient's bloodstream.

In the body, the receptors are attracted to targets on the surface of the cancer cells.

The CAR T cells identify the cancer cells with the target antigens, and kill them.

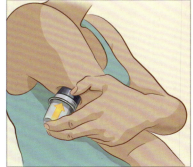
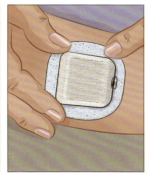
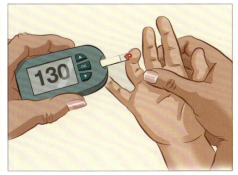
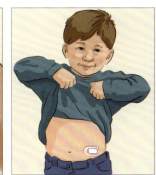

130

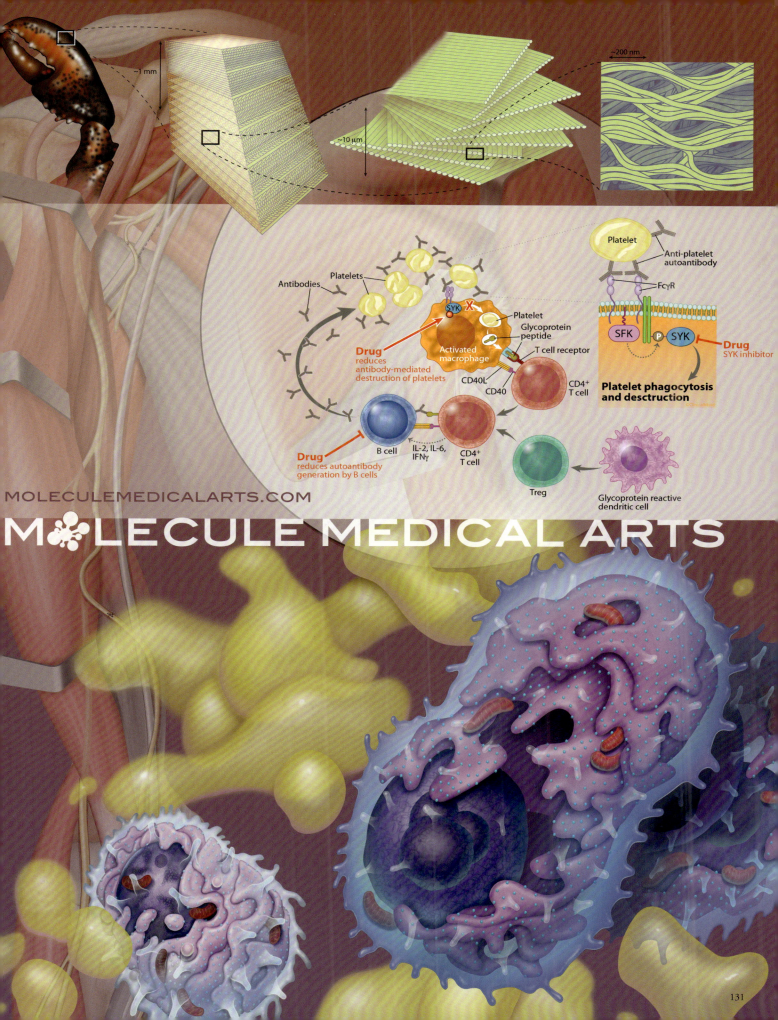

~1 mm

~10 μm

~200 nm

Antibodies

Platelets

Drug
reduces
antibody-mediated
destruction of platelets

SYK X

Activated
macrophage

Platelet

Glycoprotein
peptide

T cell receptor

CD40L

CD40

CD4+
T cell

Drug
reduces autoantibody
generation by B cells

B cell

IL-2, IL-6,
IFNγ

CD4+
T cell

Treg

Glycoprotein reactive
dendritic cell

Platelet

Anti-platelet
autoantibody

FcγR

SFK

P

SYK

Drug
SYK inhibitor

Platelet phagocytosis
and desctruction

MOLECULEMEDICALARTS.COM

MOLECULE MEDICAL ARTS

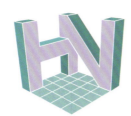

HAN NGUYEN
STUDIO

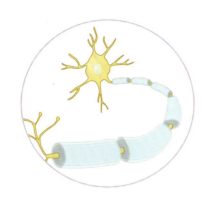

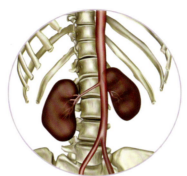

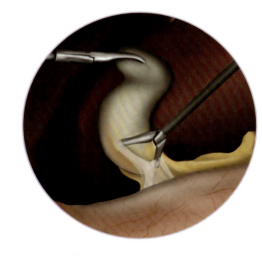

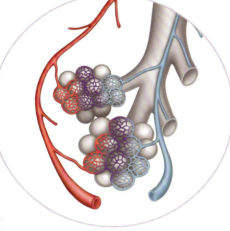

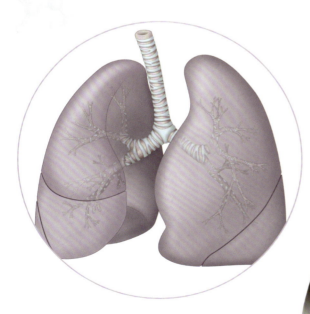

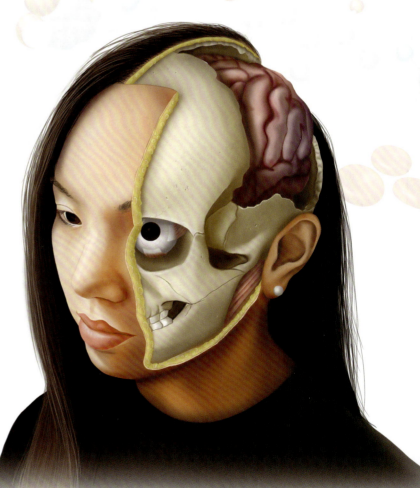

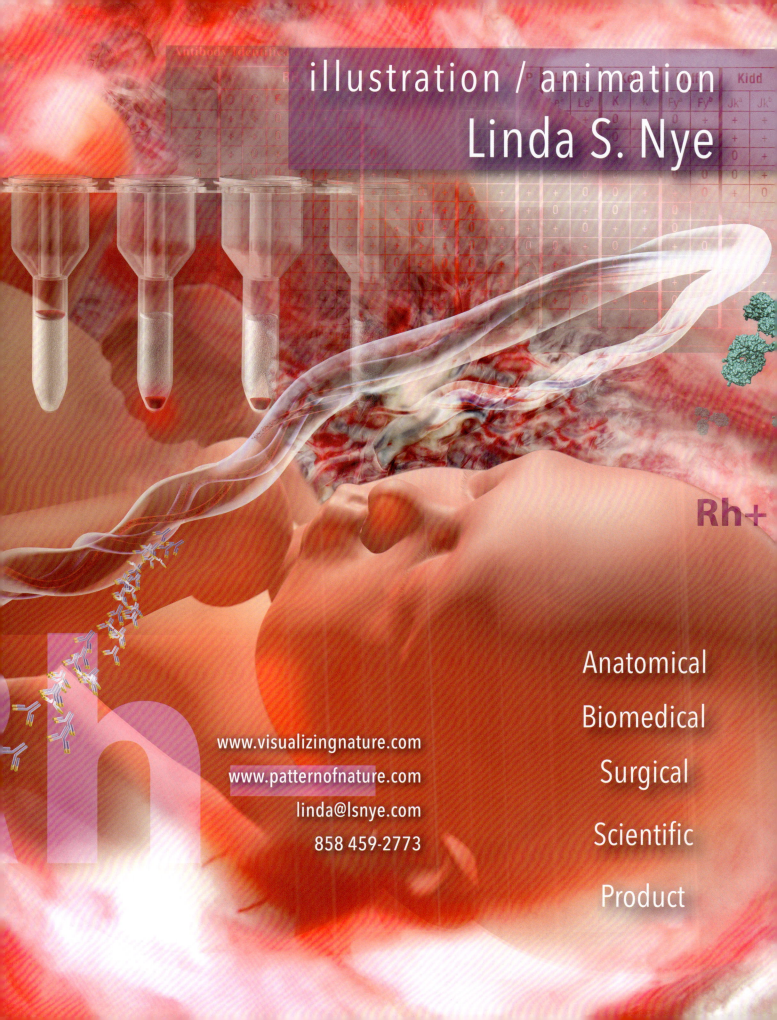

illustration / animation
Linda S. Nye

Kidd

Rh+

Anatomical

Biomedical

Surgical

Scientific

Product

www.visualizingnature.com
www.patternofnature.com
linda@lsnye.com
858 459-2773

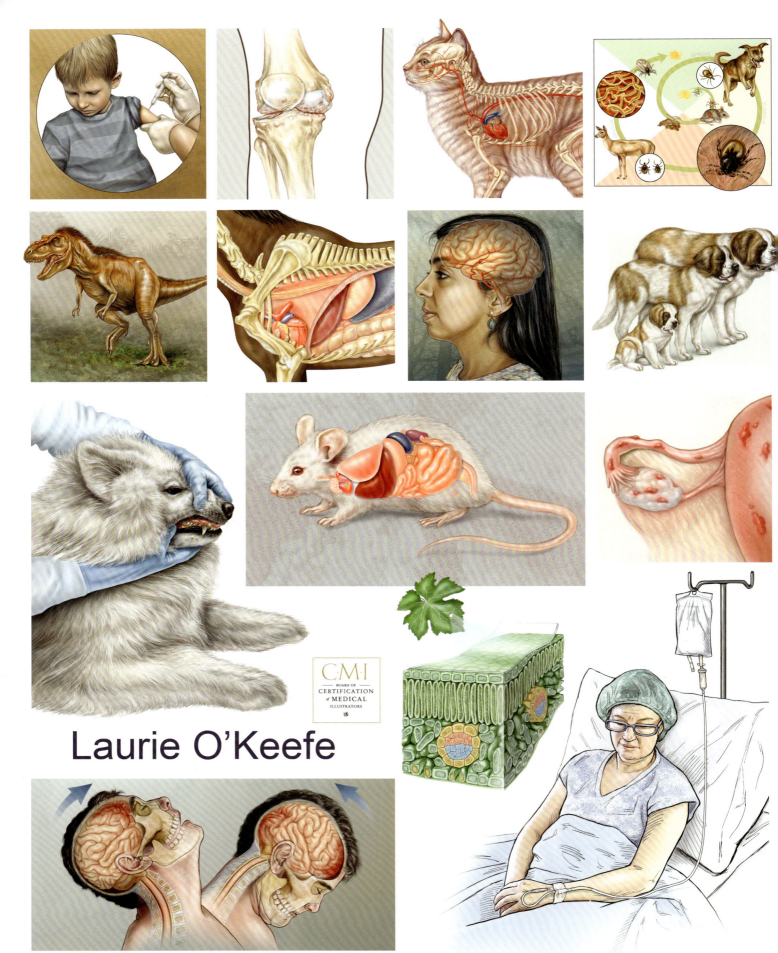

Laurie O'Keefe

laurieokeefe.com   okeefe@rockisland.com   360-303-2967

tejeswini padma

tejeswinipadma.com
tejeswini.padma@gmail.com
+919108751123

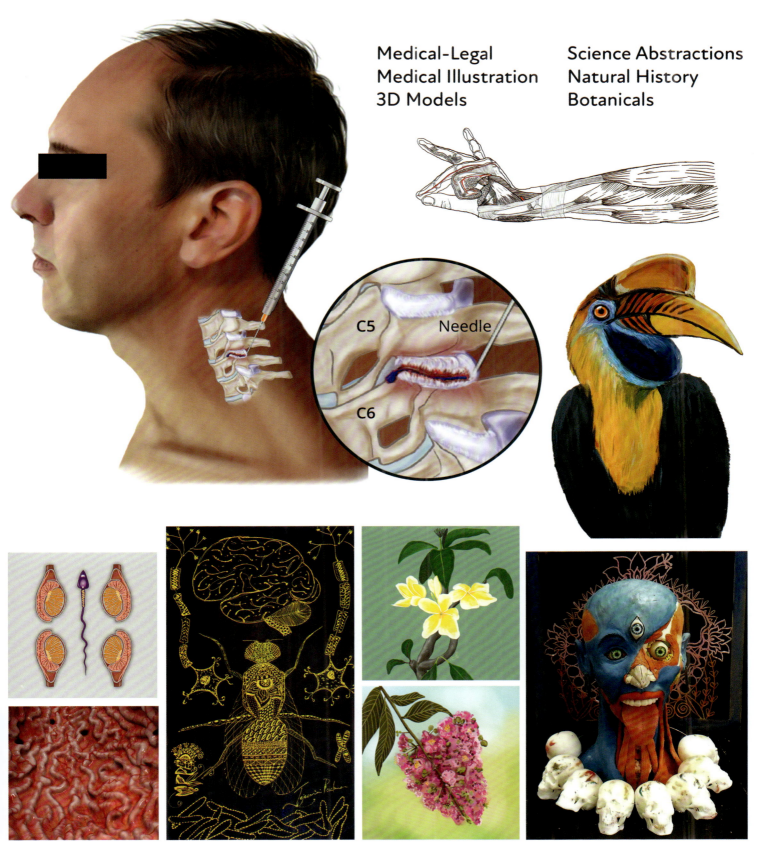

Medical-Legal
Medical Illustration
3D Models

Science Abstractions
Natural History
Botanicals

C5 Needle

C6

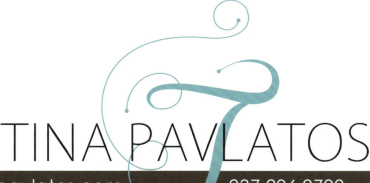

TINA PAVLATOS

www.tinapavlatos.com 937.206.9700 tina@tinapavlatos.com

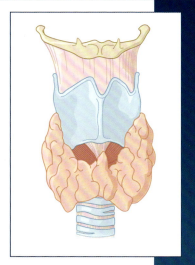

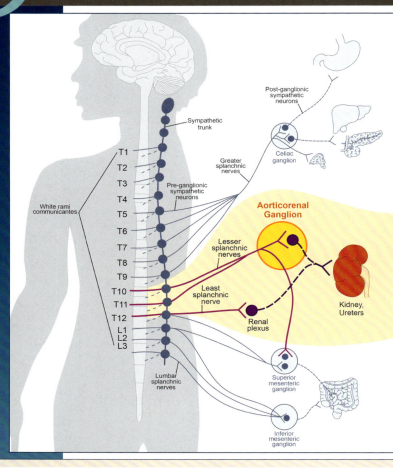

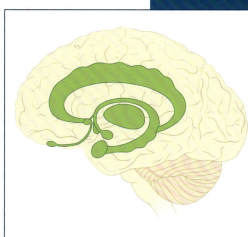

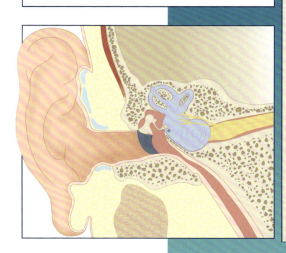

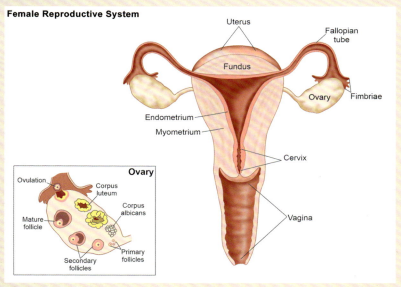

Female Reproductive System

136

Illustration•Natura

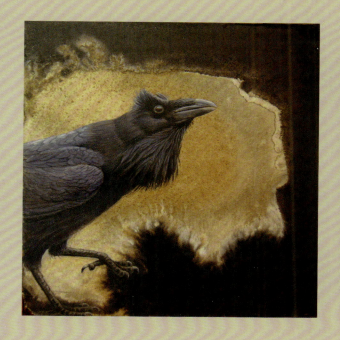

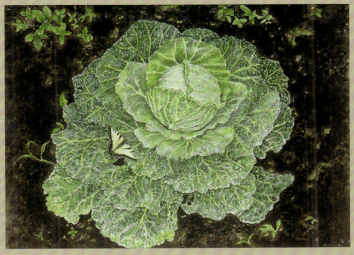

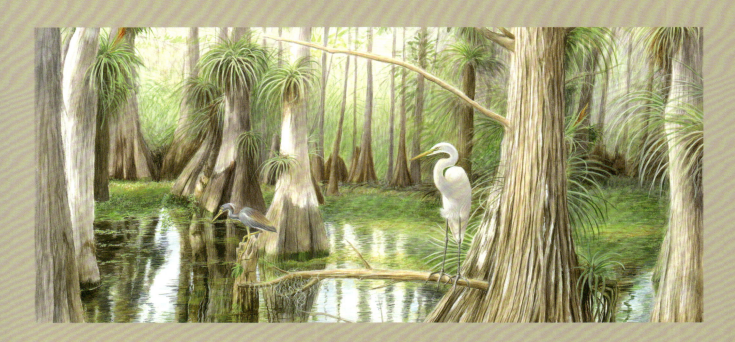

Dorie Petrochko-Studio.com

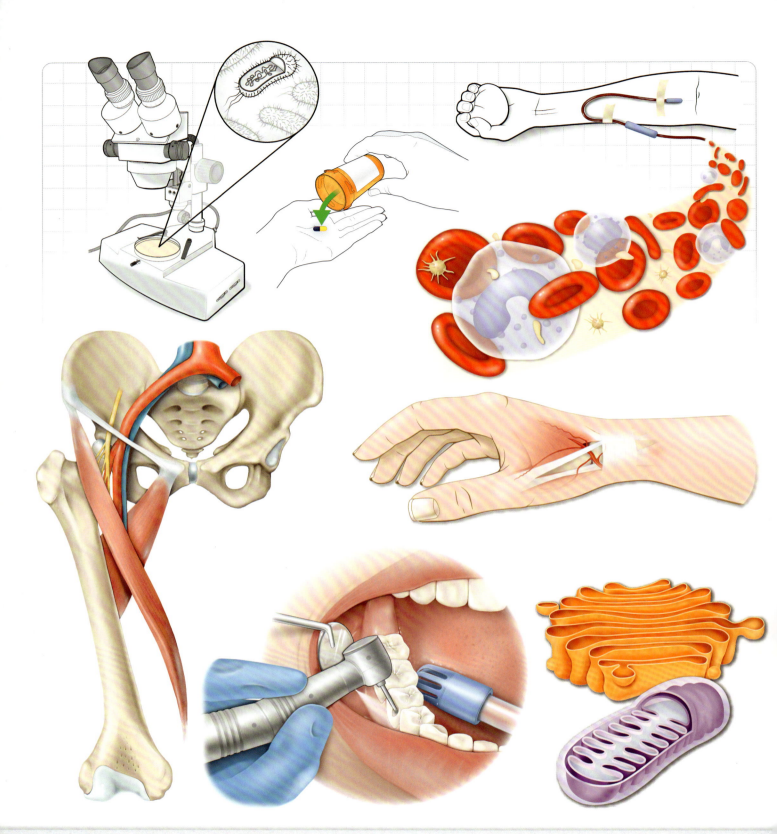

Your Ideas,
**Expressed
& Elevated**

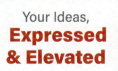
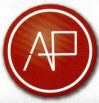

Allyson Porter
Medical and Scientific Illustration
portervisual@gmail.com   allysonportervisual.com

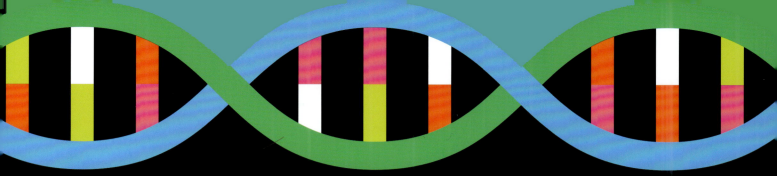

SCIENCE / MEDICINE / NATURAL HISTORY / ARCHAEOLOGY / HERITAGE

medical mission!

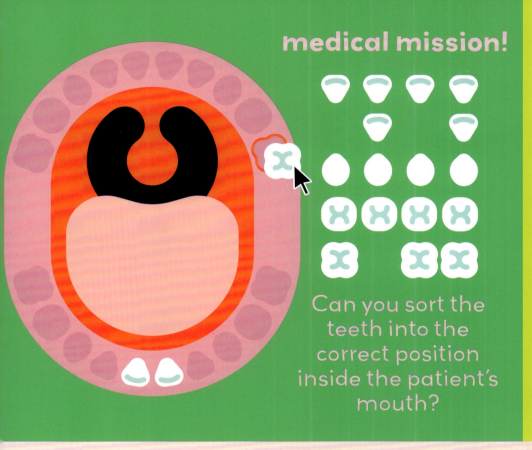

Can you sort the teeth into the correct position inside the patient's mouth?

katy potaty

BA (HONS) ILLUSTRATION

18 years experience as a digital illustrator in the UK working on:

Educational Resources
Children's E-Learning
Interactive Experiences
Workbooks & Worksheets
Editorial & Journals
Publishing
Infographics & Diagrams

www.katypotaty.co.uk
info@katypotaty.co.uk
+44(0)7919 046904

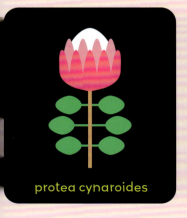

protea cynaroides

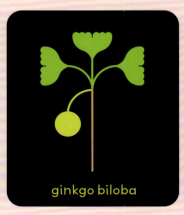

ginkgo biloba

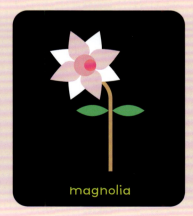

magnolia

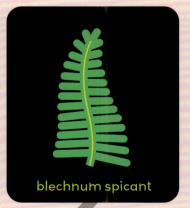

blechnum spicant

Carefully cut out the prehistoric plants and match them with the correct descriptions.

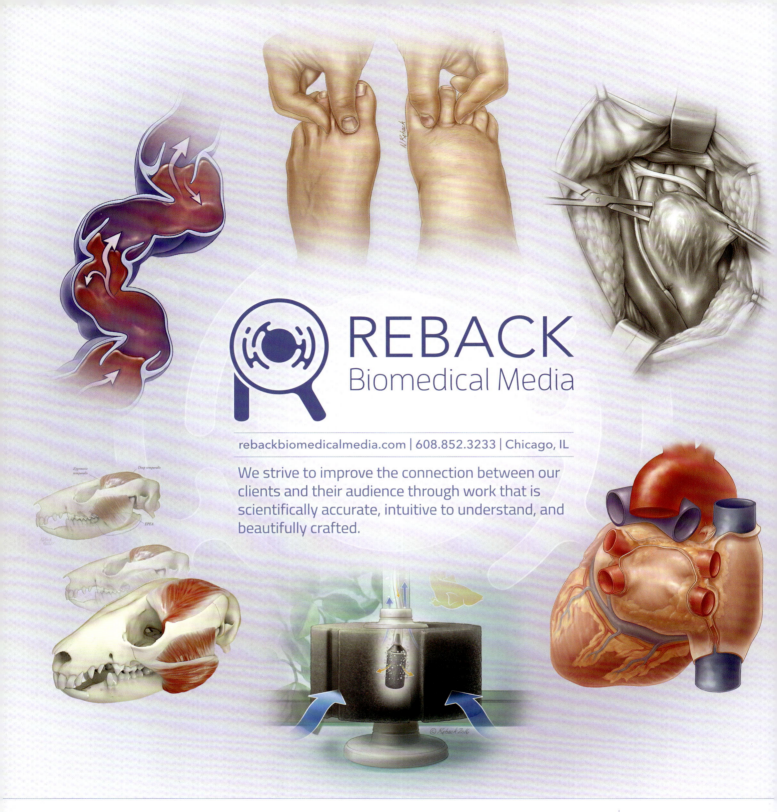

REBACK
Biomedical Media

rebackbiomedicalmedia.com | 608.852.3233 | Chicago, IL

We strive to improve the connection between our clients and their audience through work that is scientifically accurate, intuitive to understand, and beautifully crafted.

OFFERING SERVICES IN

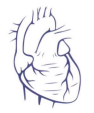

Medical illustration

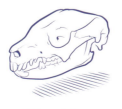

3D modeling

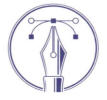

Graphic design

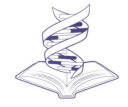

Editorial illustration

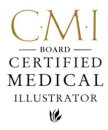

C·M·I
BOARD
CERTIFIED
MEDICAL
ILLUSTRATOR

All content © Reback Biomedical Media, 2015-2021. All rights reserved. Nicholas Reback, principal and sole proprietor.

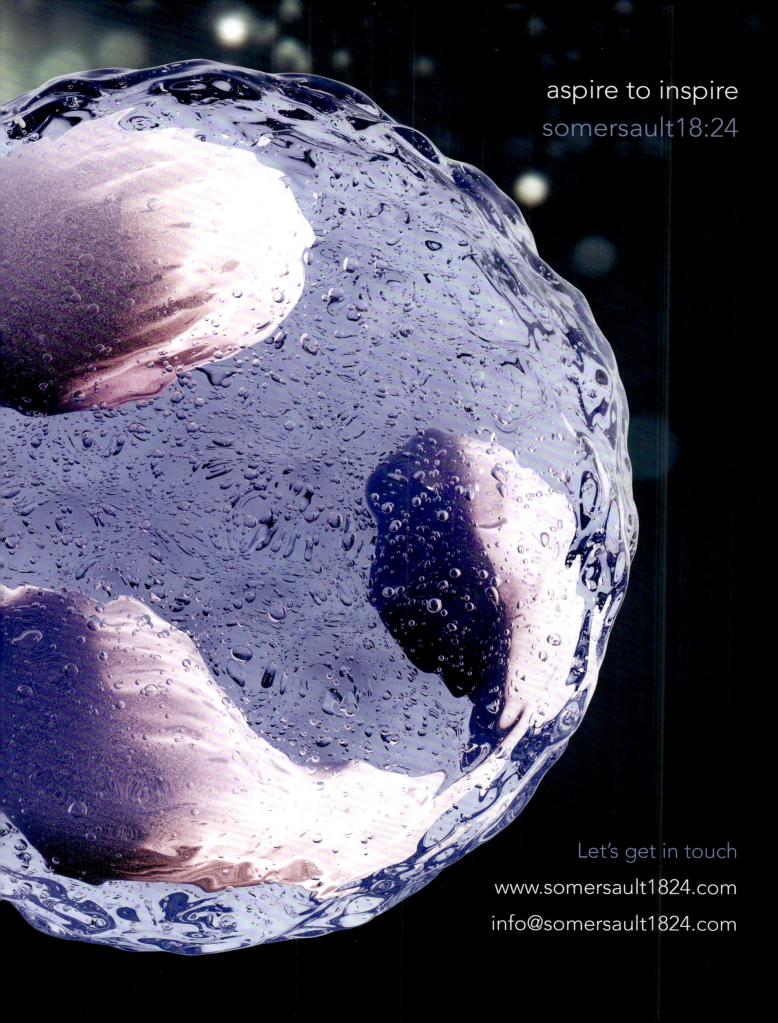

aspire to inspire
somersault18:24

Let's get in touch

www.somersault1824.com

info@somersault1824.com

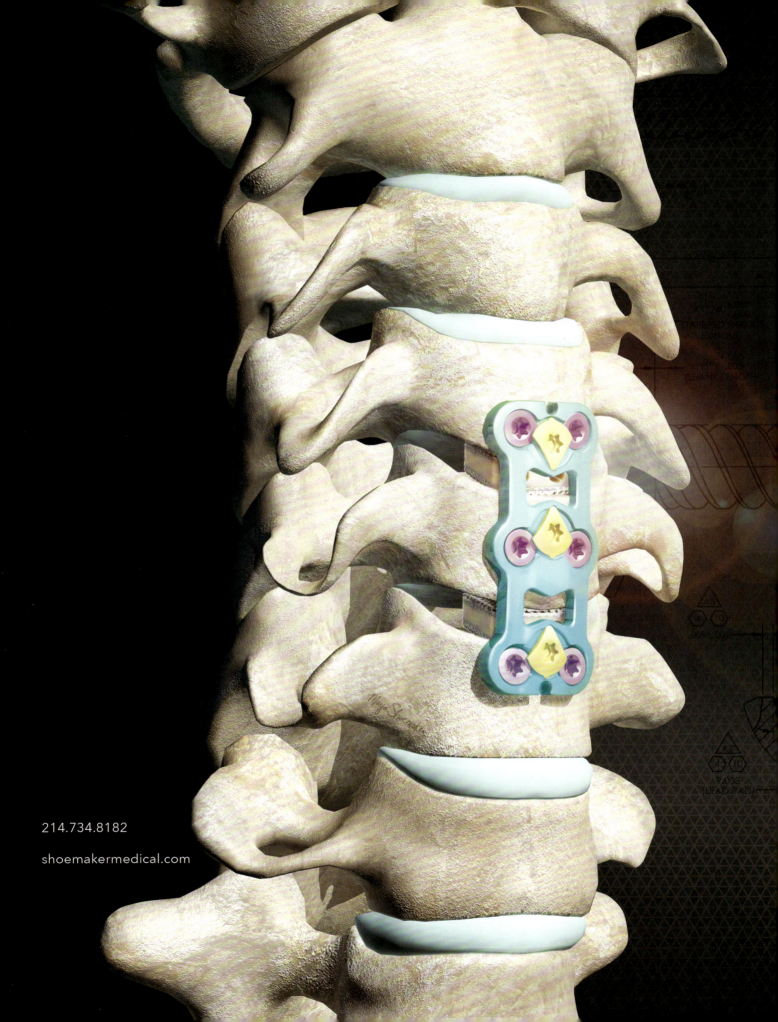

214.734.8182

shoemakermedical.com

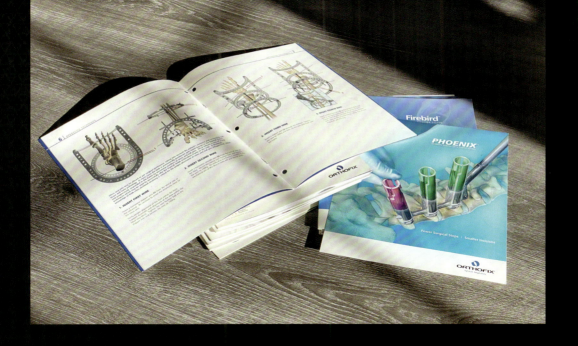

SHOEMAKER
MEDICAL

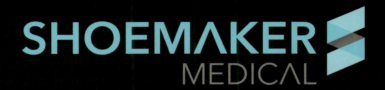

Need a surgical technique to bring a medical device to market? We can help!

Shoemaker Medical offers the accuracy you need in a beautiful package.

Illustration   Medical writing   Design

KRYSTYNA SRODULSKI

MEDICAL & SCIENTIFIC ILLUSTRATION

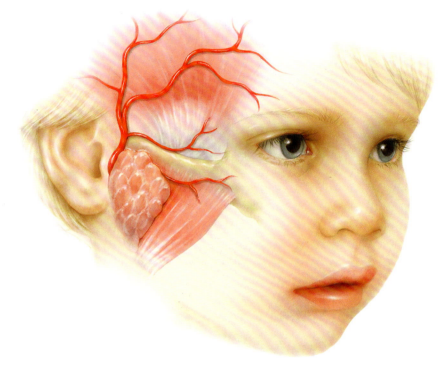

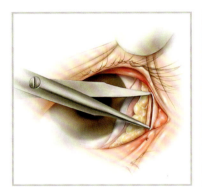

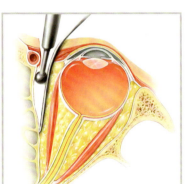

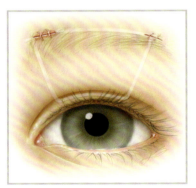

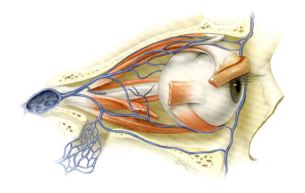

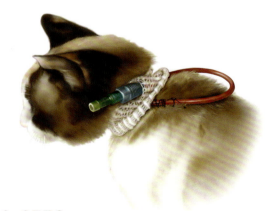

+1 (210) 862-6776

kryssrodulski@gmail.com

subQstudio

www.subqstudio.com

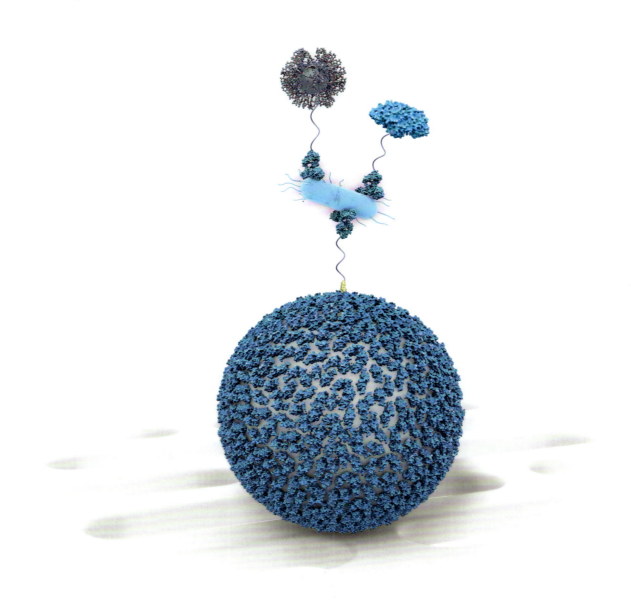

medical • surgical • biological

2d • Illustration • 3d

TETRODOTOXIN
C₁₁ H₁₇ N₃ O₈

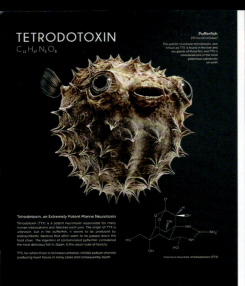

Pufferfish
(Tetrodontidae)
The potent neurotoxin tetrodotoxin, also known as TTX, is found in the liver and sex glands of these fish, and TTX is considered one of the most poisonous substances on earth.

Tetrodotoxin, an Extremely Potent Marine Neurotoxin

Tetrodotoxin (TTX) is a potent neurotoxin responsible for many human intoxications and fatalities each year. The origin of TTX is unknown, but in the pufferfish, it seems to be produced by endosymbiotic bacteria that often seem to be passed down the food chain. The ingestion of contaminated pufferfish, considered the most delicious fish in Japan, is the usual route of toxicity.

TTX, for which there is no known antidote, inhibits sodium channel producing heart failure in many cases and consequently death.

Chemical structure of tetrodotoxin (TTX)

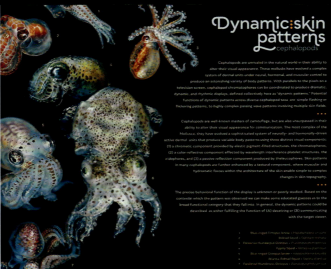

Dynamic skin patterns
cephalopods

Cephalopods are unrivaled in the natural world in their ability to alter their visual appearance. These mollusks have evolved a complex system of dermal units under neural, hormonal, and muscular control to produce an astonishing variety of body patterns. With parallels to the pixels on a television screen, cephalopod chromatophores can be coordinated to produce dramatic, dynamic, and rhythmic displays, defined collectively here as "dynamic patterns." Potential functions of dynamic patterns across diverse cephalopod taxa are simple flashing or flickering patterns, to highly complex passing wave patterns involving multiple skin fields.

Cephalopods are well-known masters of camouflage, but are also unsurpassed in their ability to alter their visual appearance for communication. The most complex of the Mollusca, they have evolved a sophisticated system of neurally- and hormonally-driven active dermal units that produce variable body patterns using three distinct visual components: (1) a chromatic component provided by elastic pigment-filled structures, the chromatophores, (2) a color-reflective component effected by wavelength interference platelet structures, the iridophores, and (3) a passive reflection component produced by the leucophores. Skin patterns in many cephalopods are further enhanced by a textural component, where muscular and hydrostatic forces within the architecture of the skin enable simple to complex changes in skin topography.

The precise behavioral function of the display is unknown or poorly studied. Based on the context in which the pattern was observed we can make some educated guesses as to the broad functional category that they fall into. In general, the dynamic patterns could be described as either fulfilling the function of (A) deceiving or (B) communicating with the target viewer.

Axolotl_ambystoma mexicanum_

Conservation status

extinct		threatened			least concern	
EX	EW	CR	EN	VU	NT	LC

Critically Endangered

Scientific classification

Kingdom:	Animalia
Phylum:	Chordata
Class:	Amphibia
Order:	Urodela
Family:	Ambystomatidae
Genus:	Ambystoma
Species:	A. mexicanum

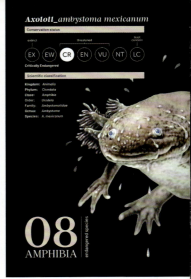

08
AMPHIBIA
endangered species

SILK WORM
{*Bombyx mori*}

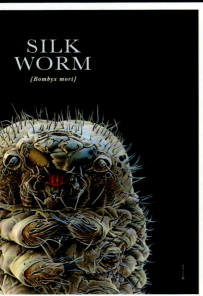

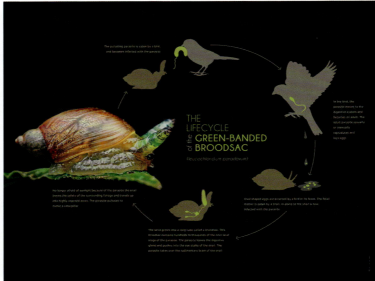

THE LIFECYCLE of the
GREEN-BANDED BROODSAC
(Leucochloridium paradoxum)

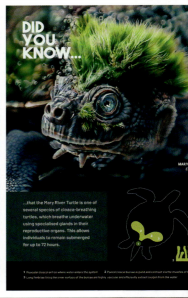

DID YOU KNOW...

...that the Mary River Turtle is one of several species of cloaca-breathing turtles, which breathe underwater using specialised glands in their reproductive organs. This allows individuals to remain submerged for up to 72 hours.

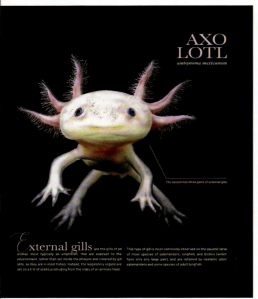

AXO LOTL
ambystoma mexicanum

The axolotl has four pairs of external gills

External gills are the gills of an animal, most typically an amphibian, that are exposed to the environment, rather than set inside the pharynx and covered by gill slits, as they are in most fishes. Instead, the respiratory organs are set on a frill of stalks protruding from the sides of an animal's head.

This type of gill is most commonly observed on the aquatic larva of most species of salamanders, lungfish, and bichirs (which have only one large pair), and are retained by neotenic adult salamanders and some species of adult lungfish.

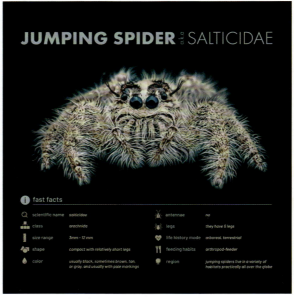

JUMPING SPIDER aka SALTICIDAE

ⓘ fast facts

scientific name	salticidae	antennae	no
class	arachnida	legs	they have 8 legs
size range	3mm - 12 mm	life history mode	arboreal, terrestrial
shape	compact with relatively short legs	feeding habits	arthropod-feeder
color	usually black, sometimes brown, tan, or gray, and usually with pale markings	region	jumping spiders live in a variety of habitats practically all over the globe

---

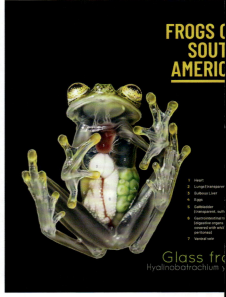

FROGS OF SOUTH AMERICA

1 Heart
2 Lungs (transparent...)
3 Bulbous Liver
4 Eggs
5 Gallbladder (transparent, sulf...)
6 Gastrointestinal t... (digestive organs... covered with whit... peritoneal)
7 Ventral vein

Glass frog
Hyalinobatrachium...

Studio Lindalu

studiolindalu.com
info@studiolindalu.com
@studio.lindalu

Scientific Visualization | Illustration | Graphic Design

 by Linda Lubbersen

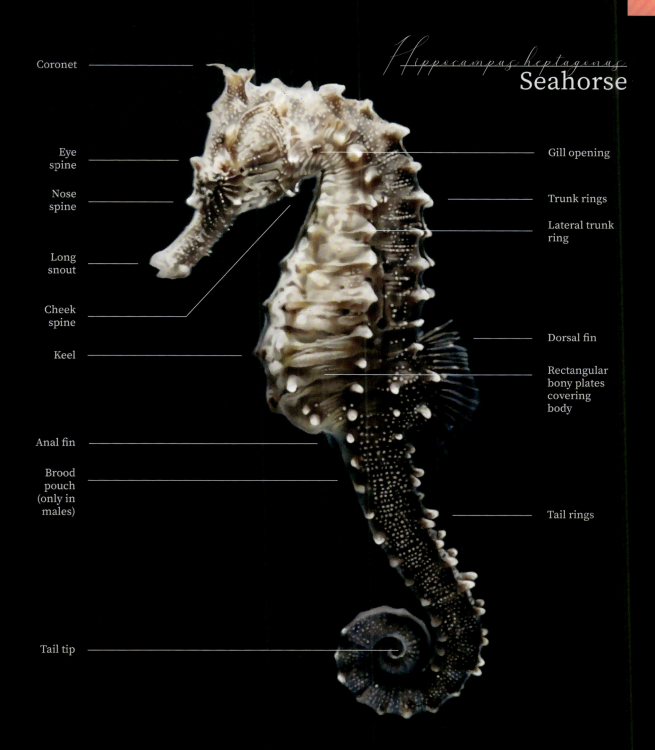

Coronet

Hippocampus heptagonus
Seahorse

Eye
spine

Gill opening

Nose
spine

Trunk rings

Lateral trunk
ring

Long
snout

Cheek
spine

Keel

Dorsal fin

Rectangular
bony plates
covering
body

Anal fin

Brood
pouch
(only in
males)

Tail rings

Tail tip

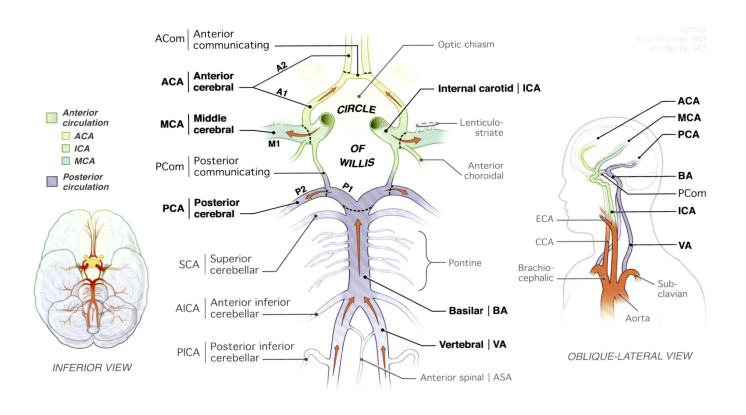

Anterior communicating | ACom

Anterior cerebral | ACA

A2

A1

Middle cerebral | MCA

M1

Posterior communicating | PCom

Posterior cerebral | PCA

P2 P1

Superior cerebellar | SCA

Anterior inferior cerebellar | AICA

Posterior inferior cerebellar | PICA

Optic chiasm

CIRCLE OF WILLIS

Internal carotid | ICA

Lenticulo-striate

Anterior choroidal

Pontine

Basilar | BA

Vertebral | VA

Anterior spinal | ASA

Anterior circulation
- ACA
- ICA
- MCA

Posterior circulation

INFERIOR VIEW

ACA
MCA
PCA
BA
PCom
ICA
VA

ECA
CCA
Brachio-cephalic
Sub-clavian
Aorta

OBLIQUE-LATERAL VIEW

ANDREA CHAREST
Chicago

THIRD LEFT STUDIOS
→ Images with Direction

KARINA METCALF
Los Angeles

www.thirdleftstudios.com | info@thirdleftstudios.com

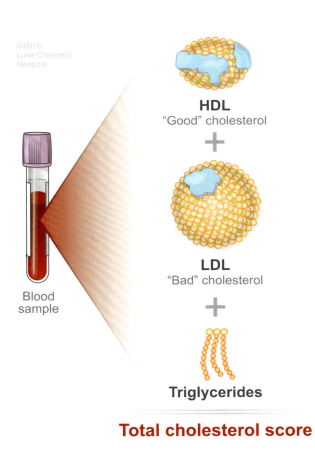

HDL
"Good" cholesterol

+

LDL
"Bad" cholesterol

+

Triglycerides

Total cholesterol score

Blood sample

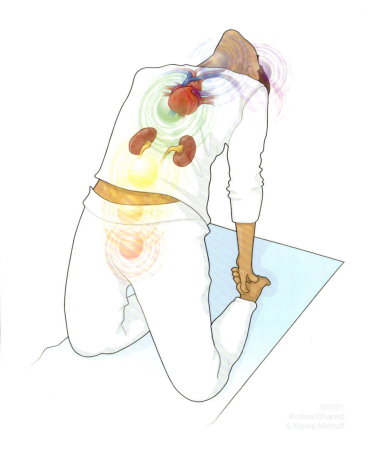

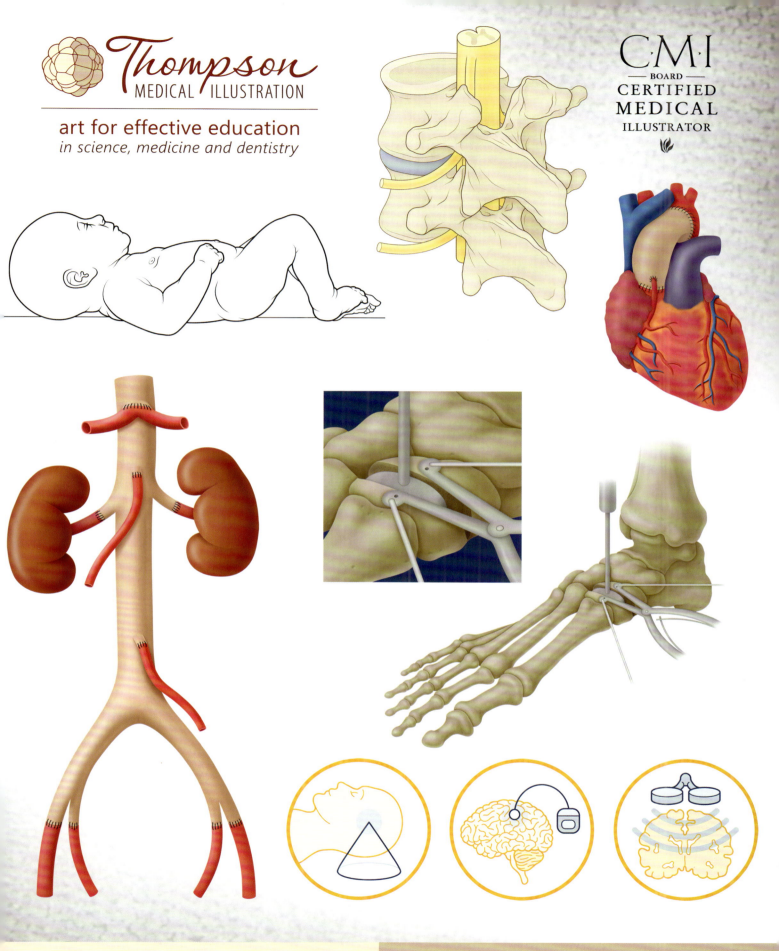

Molly Thompson, CMI | Pittsburgh, PA   tmillustration.com | 412.353.9278

VISUALIZING SCIENCE

Custom Solutions
For visual communication

- infographics
- illustrations
- data visualization
- motion graphics
- layout design with 508 compliance

CASE STUDY

rough sketches

Tailored Styles
To fit your audience and your brand

- clean vector
- pen-and-ink
- watercolor or acrylic
- typography

Recent testimonial:

"As usual, [Fiona] delved into the science, lifted out what's important, and designed a creative, high-quality product."

—REBECCA LINDSEY, NOAA

preliminary

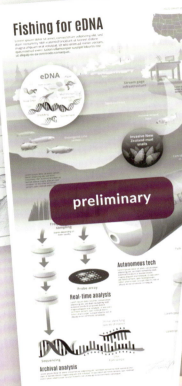

Fiona makes changes at each stage following scientists' advice.

final rendering

Art by Fiona Martin of Visualizing Science, © 2021 MBARI

follow

Fiona Martin
Creative Director ▪ Scientific Illustrator ▪ Designer

www.visualizingscience.com

480-414-0301 ▪ fiona@visualizingscience.com

scan

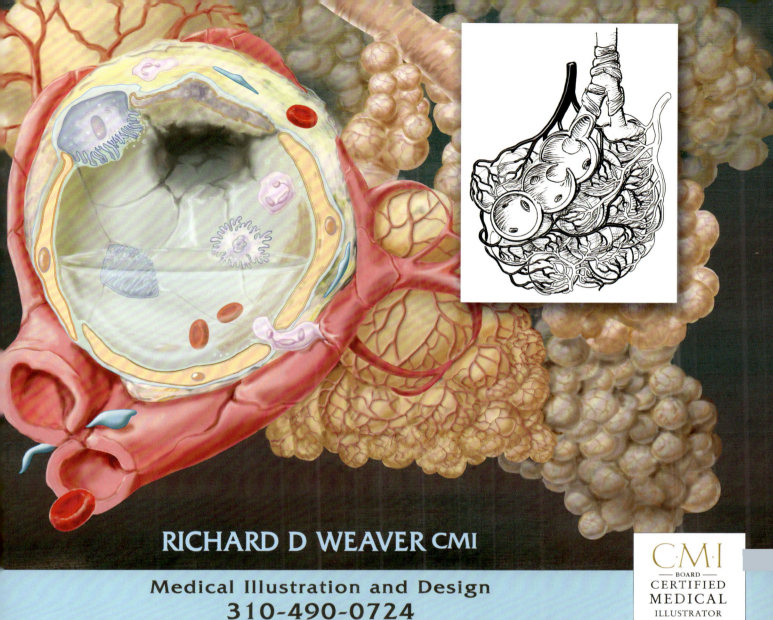

RICHARD D WEAVER CMI

Medical Illustration and Design
310-490-0724
18 East Ridge Court • Parachute, Colorado • 81635
rdweaver@earthlink.net • www. DWeaverDesigns.com

C·M·I
— BOARD —
CERTIFIED
MEDICAL
ILLUSTRATOR

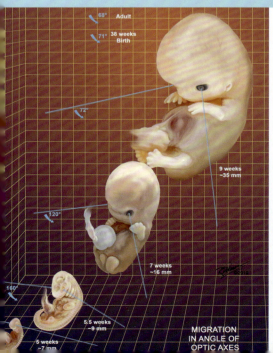

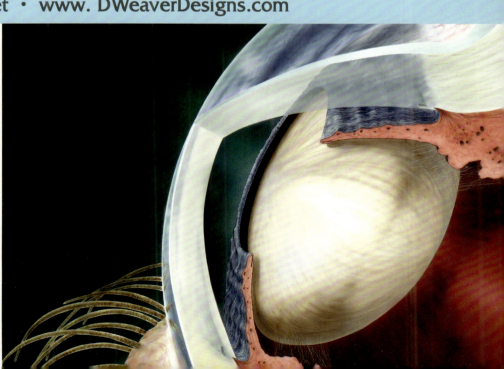

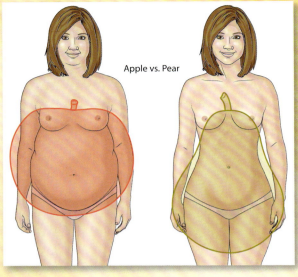

Apple vs. Pear

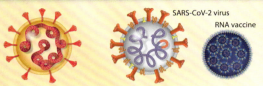

SARS-CoV-2 virus

RNA vaccine

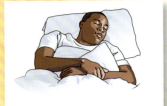

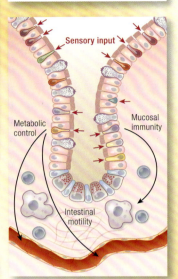

Sensory input

Metabolic control

Mucosal immunity

Intestinal motility

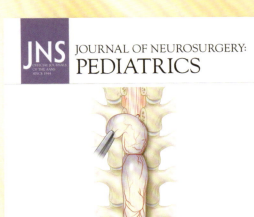

JNS — OFFICIAL JOURNALS OF THE AANS SINCE 1944

JOURNAL OF NEUROSURGERY: PEDIATRICS

June 2020
Volume 25
Number 6
www.thejns.org

The American Society of Pediatric Neurosurgeons

American Association of Neurological Surgeons

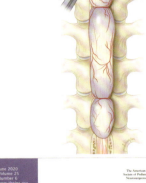

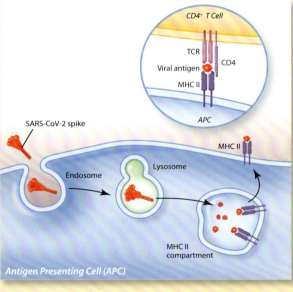

CD4⁺ T Cell

$CD4^+$ T Cell

TCR

CD4

Viral antigen

MHC II

APC

SARS-CoV-2 spike

Endosome

Lysosome

MHC II

MHC II compartment

Antigen Presenting Cell (APC)

C·M·I
— BOARD —
CERTIFIED
MEDICAL
ILLUSTRATOR

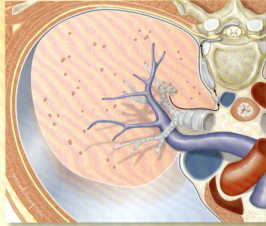

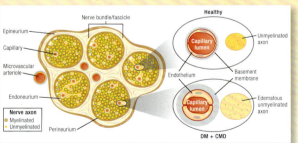

Nerve bundle/fascicle

Healthy

Epineurium

Capillary

Microvascular arteriole

Capillary lumen

Unmyelinated axon

Endothelium

Basement membrane

Endoneurium

Capillary lumen

Edematous unmyelinated axon

Perineurium

Nerve axon
- Myelinated
- Unmyelinated

DM + CMD

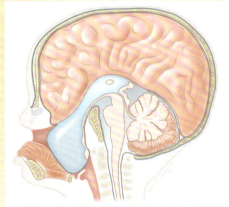

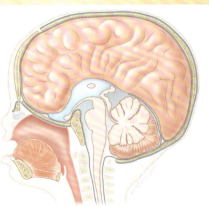

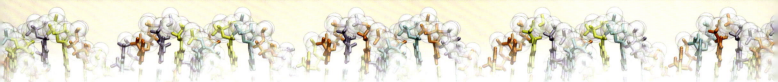

Jane Whitney B.Sc. A.A.M. CMI

www.janewhitney.com

Medical & Scientific Illustrator
416-264-2493

What follows is but a glimpse into the depth and breadth of contributions made by Medical Illustrators to illuminate the science of the COVID-19 global pandemic.

We are honored to thank and pay tribute to them here in this historic edition.

Medical illustrators raced to collaborate with researchers to help uncover the structure of the novel coronavirus COVID-19, then worked and re-worked artistic concepts as new science emerged. We helped explain the virus's mechanism of infection and how to prevent its spread. We partnered with innovators to patent new types of PPE, explained how the vaccine candidates work, and re-conceptualized health care spaces to better accommodate highly infectious patient populations. This was a massive community undertaking to educate the public and attempt to save lives.

— RACHEL BAJEMA
An Historic Year for Medical Illustration

View artist portfolios online at

MEDILLSB.COM

COVID-19 ARTISTS TRIBUTE

View artist portfolios online at

MEDILLSB.COM

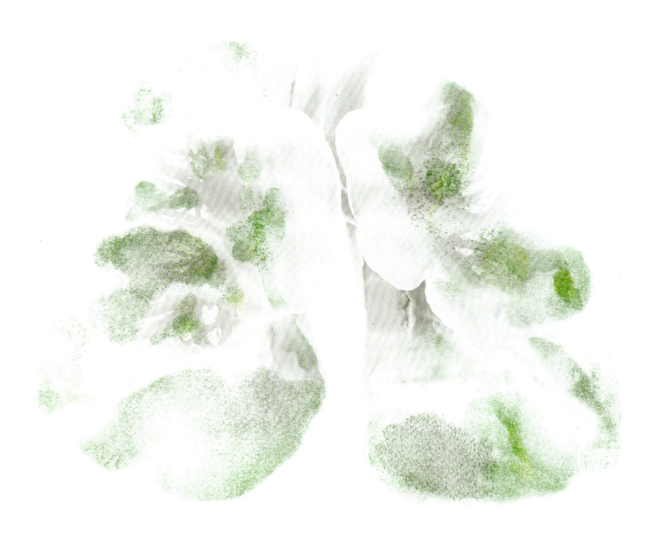

Bajema Studios

page 18

bajemastudios.com

COVID-19 Infection in the Lungs

This piece is an artistic visualization of COVID-19 in the lungs. COVID-19 may cause the respiratory system to become inflamed, causing difficulty breathing. Severe cases may lead to pneumonia, progressing to Acute Respiratory Distress Syndrome (ARDS), a type of lung failure.

© Bajemastudios, LLC

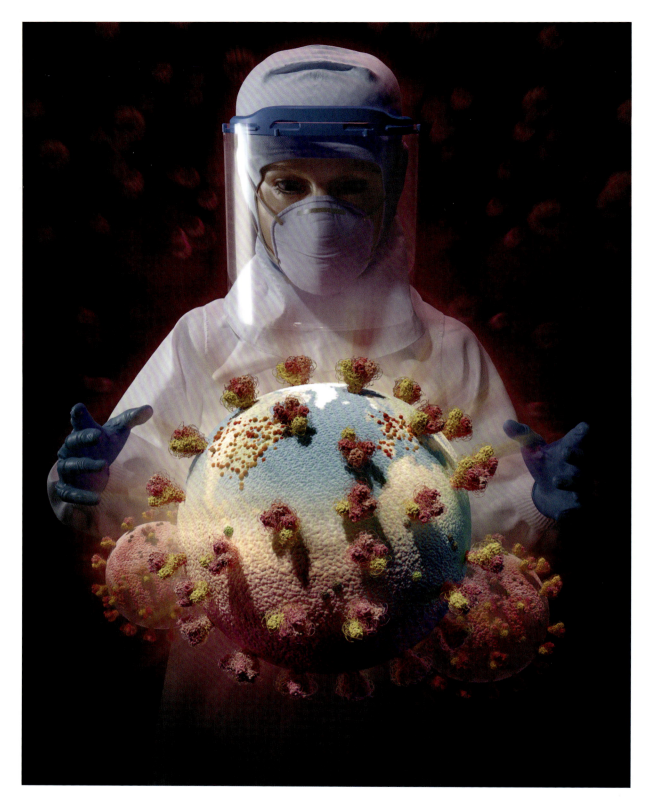

RAYMOND NELSEN
page 45

Raymond Nelsen Illustration
raymondnelsen.com

COVID-19 Earth
Illustration of the extent and impact of COVID-19.

© Raymond Nelsen Illustration

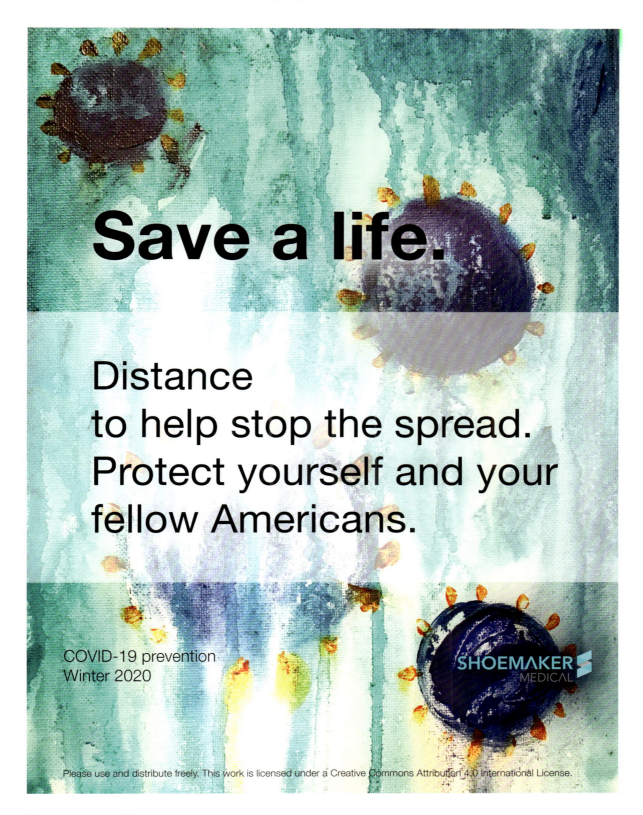

SHOEMAKER MEDICAL

page 142-143

shoemakermedical.com

COVID-19 Poster Series

One in a series of posters promoting public behaviors to prevent the spread of COVID-19.

© Maya Shoemaker, 2020

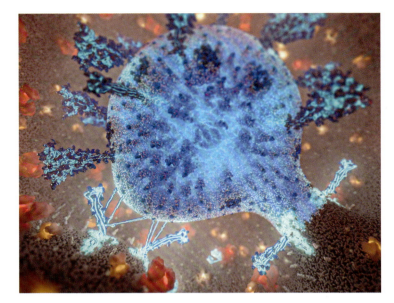

3-D.SCIENCE *(left)*
page 9

3-D.science

A SARS-CoV-2 virion infects a cell.

© Dr. Christoph Kuehne

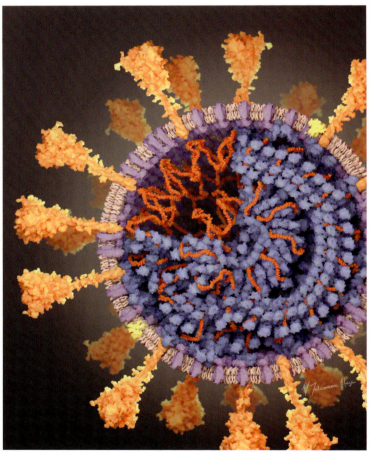

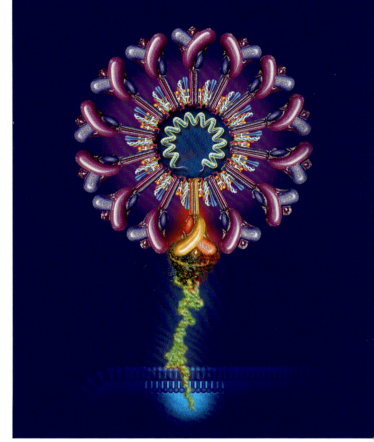

VERONICA FALCONIERI HAYS *(above)*

Falconieri Visuals
falconierivisuals.com

SARS-CoV-2 Virion in 3D

3D model of SARS-CoV-2 virion structure (based on knowledge of SARS-CoV-2 structures as of April, 2020)

© 2020 Veronica Falconieri Hays.

JOE CHOVAN *(above)*
page 82-83

Healthcare Visuals
www.medillsb.com/joechovan

COV-19 and Cell Receptor

Published in *JACC (Journals of American College of Cardiology): Basic to Translational Science* where it helped to describe the process of the virus infecting the human cell.

© Joe Chovan

COVID-19

Is a disease caused by the virus SARS-CoV-2 that can cause lethal illness and spread from person to person.

1 A virus enters the cells of the eyes, nose and mouth through the air or touch.

2 Each virus makes copies of itself. This destroys the cell and allows the virus to spread to other cells.

3 Destroyed cells and large amounts of virus activate the immune system, causing inflammation and symptoms.

4 Inflamed alveolar sacs need to work harder to provide oxygen to the blood that circulates throughout the body.

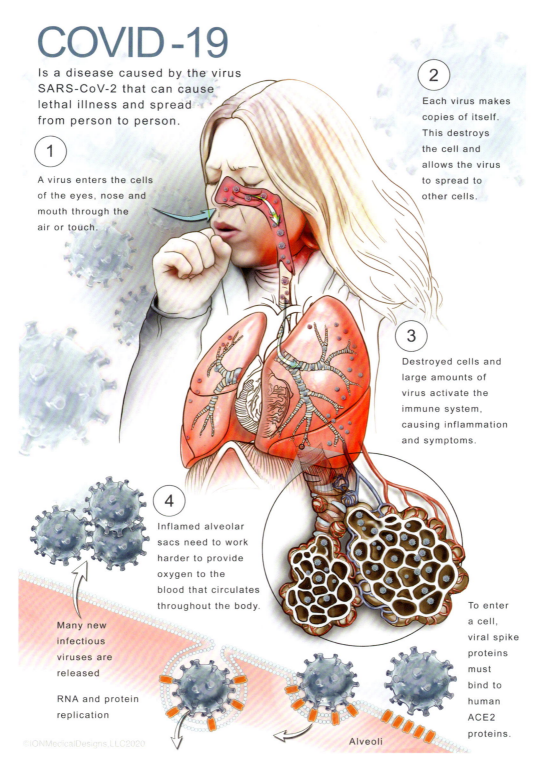

Many new infectious viruses are released

RNA and protein replication

©IONMedicalDesigns,LLC2020

To enter a cell, viral spike proteins must bind to human ACE2 proteins.

Alveoli

LINDSAY COULTER

ION Medical Designs, LLC
www.ionmedicaldesigns.com

Public Education Illustration

This illustration was created to help educate the general public on how COVID-19 is contracted, travels to the respiratory tract and reproduces in the aveolar cells.

© ION Medical Designs, LLC

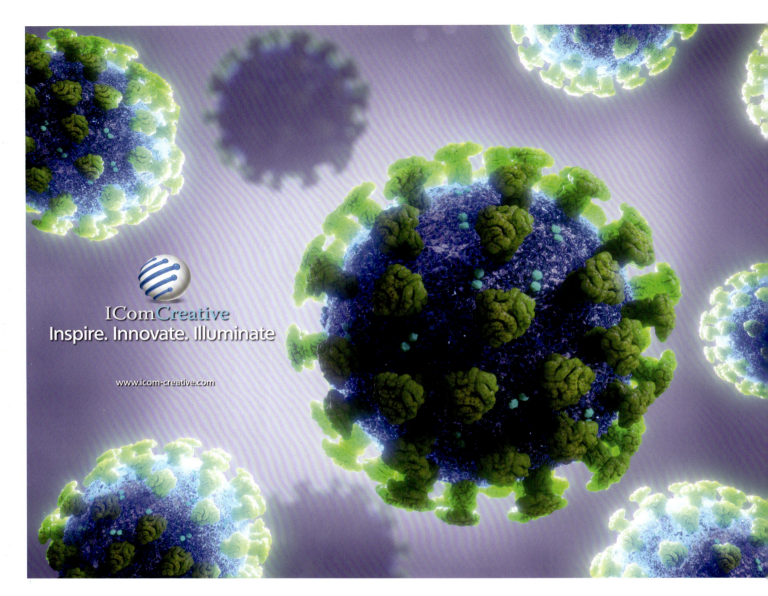

ICom Creative Corp *(above)*
page 36-37

icom-creative.com

Corona Virus - B.1.1.7 Variant

© ICom Creative, ICOM CREATIVE CORP

Ni-ka Ford *(right)*

Icahn School of Medicine at Mount Sinai
nikaford.com

Lungs Infected with COVID-19

This illustration depicts the cascade of events that happen on a cellular level within the lungs when they have been infected by SARS-CoV-2 or COVID-19 in severe cases.

© 2020 Mount Sinai Health System

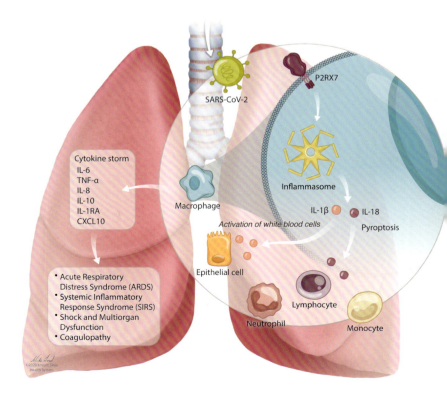

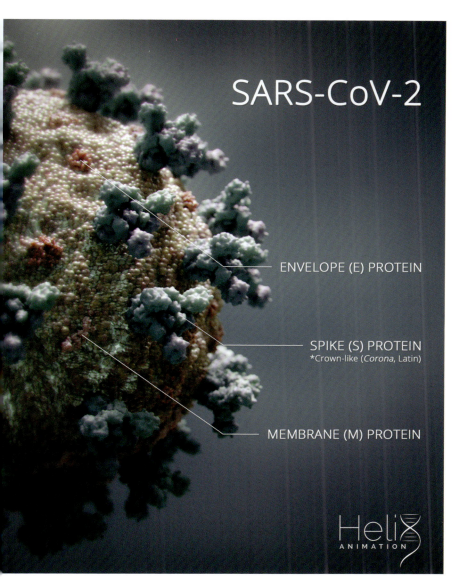

SARS-CoV-2

ENVELOPE (E) PROTEIN

SPIKE (S) PROTEIN
*Crown-like (*Corona*, Latin)

MEMBRANE (M) PROTEIN

Helix
ANIMATION

HELIX ANIMATION *(left)*
page 32-33

helixanimation.com

3D Stylized Visualization of COVID-19

This piece highlights the most common means of COVID-19 transmission, and an artistic representation of the SARS-CoV-2 virus that causes it.

© Helix Animation 2020. All Rights Reserved

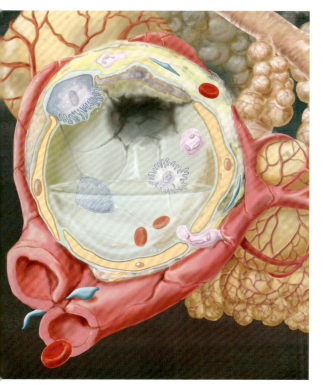

RICHARD WEAVER *(left)*
page 151

DWeaver Designs
dweaverdesigns.com

Covid-19-infected Aveolus, Detail.

This piece illustrates injuries in aveolus occurring during the acute phase of SARS-CoV-2 infection. The image opens a view inside one sac showing intact and dying Type II epithelial cells, adjacent to necrotic type I cells (gray), and an aveolar macrophage. The interior of the globe is half-filled with protein-rich fluid as the protective surfactant layer inactivates and a hyaline membrane forms. The enmeshing capillaries are weakened, leaking neutrophils, fibroblasts and RBCs into the interior.

© Richard D Weaver, CMI

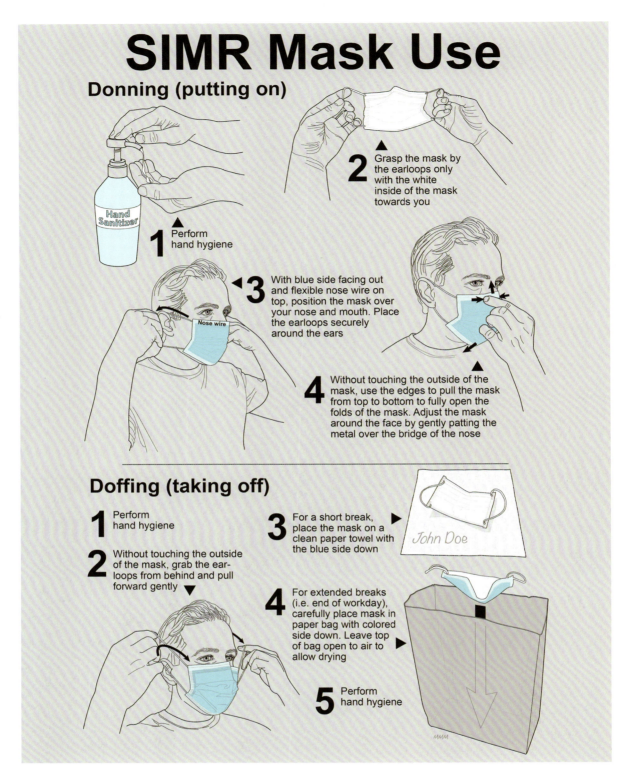

SIMR Mask Use

Donning (putting on)

1 Perform hand hygiene

2 Grasp the mask by the earloops only with the white inside of the mask towards you

3 With blue side facing out and flexible nose wire on top, position the mask over your nose and mouth. Place the earloops securely around the ears

4 Without touching the outside of the mask, use the edges to pull the mask from top to bottom to fully open the folds of the mask. Adjust the mask around the face by gently patting the metal over the bridge of the nose

Doffing (taking off)

1 Perform hand hygiene

2 Without touching the outside of the mask, grab the earloops from behind and pull forward gently

3 For a short break, place the mask on a clean paper towel with the blue side down

John Doe

4 For extended breaks (i.e. end of workday), carefully place mask in paper bag with colored side down. Leave top of bag open to air to allow drying

5 Perform hand hygiene

MARK MILLER
STOWERS INSTITUTE

Stowers Institute for Medical Research
Miller Medical Illustration
millermedart.com

SIMR (Stowers Institute for Medical Research) Mask Use

Line art with color showing the proper steps of donning and doffing a mask. The poster format is displayed internally at multiple locations.

© Mark M. Miller © SIMR

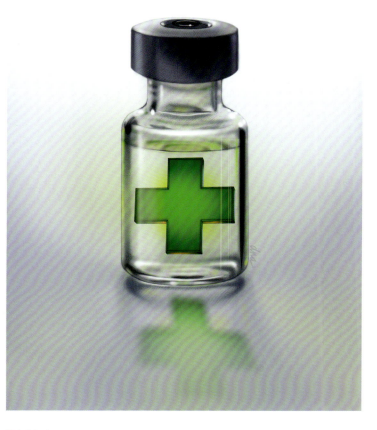

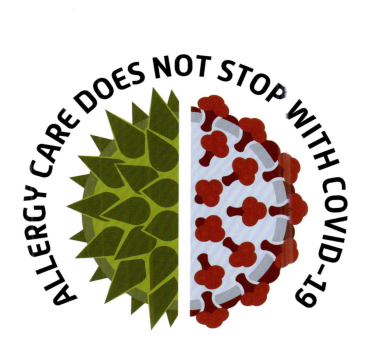

DNA Illustrations *(above)*
page 90

www.dnaillustrations.com

Hyperrealistic Rendering of a Vaccine Bottle

Cover illustration for *The Pharmaceutical Journal*, used by the Royal Pharmaceutical Society to promote the role pharmacies play in COVID vaccination in the largest immunization program in the UK's history.

© DNA Illustrations

Mica Duran *(above)*
page 92-93

Mica Duran Studio
micaduran.com

World Allergy Week Campaign

Logo commissioned by the International World Allergy Organization to promote their 2020 World Allergy Week campaign, which combined messaging on allergy care and COVID-19 during the pandemic.

© 2020 Mica Duran

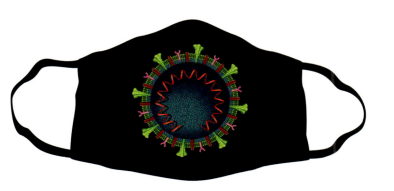

Graham Studios *(left)*
page 100

grahamstudios.net

COVID Cross-section with Black Mask

This illustration of a COVID cross-section with black mask was used as a message on social media.

© Graham Studios

161

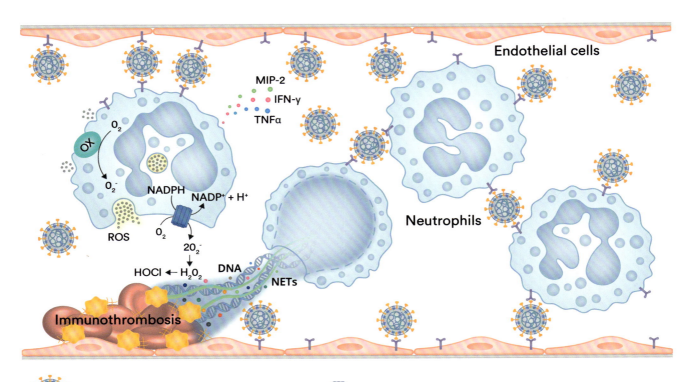

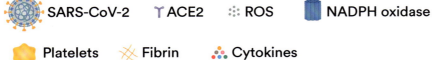

SARS-CoV-2   **Y ACE2**   **⠿ ROS**   **NADPH oxidase**

Platelets   **Fibrin**   **Cytokines**

KOLD DESIGN *(above)*

page 120

kold.design

Immunological Response to SARS-CoV-2 Infection

The SARs-CoV2 virus may be attached to neutrophils (via ACE2 receptors). This could result in a cytokine storm and the production of reactive oxygen species (ROS), inducing the release of NETs.

© 2021 KOLD DESIGN

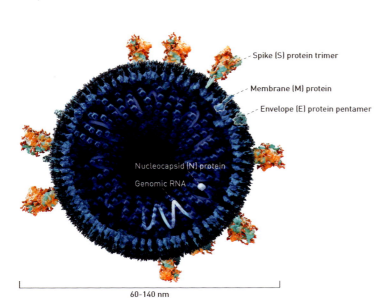

Spike (S) protein trimer

Membrane (M) protein

Envelope (E) protein pentamer

Nucleocapsid (N) protein

Genomic RNA

60-140 nm

COGNITION STUDIO, INC. *(left)*

cognitionstudio.com

Anatomy of SARS-CoV-2

Understanding SARS-CoV-2 evolved into a cross-team initiative involving science storytelling, design, writing and development. Our aim: translate complexity for knowledge translation. Client: The world.

© 2020-2021, Cognition Studio, Inc. All rights reserved.

the fight

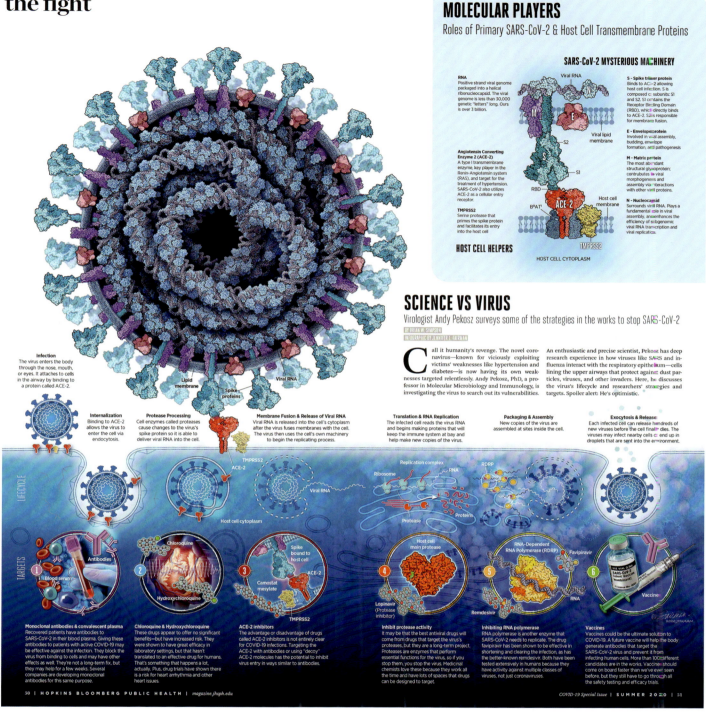

JENNIFER FAIRMAN

page 91

Johns Hopkins University, Dept. of Art As Applied to Medicine
medicalart.johnshopkins.edu/fairman

Science vs. Virus

This infographic depicts the SARS-CoV-2 virus, it's replication cycle and targeted therapies against COVID-19.

Illustration: Jennifer E. Fairman, MA, MPS, CMI, FAMI, © 2020, Johns Hopkins University

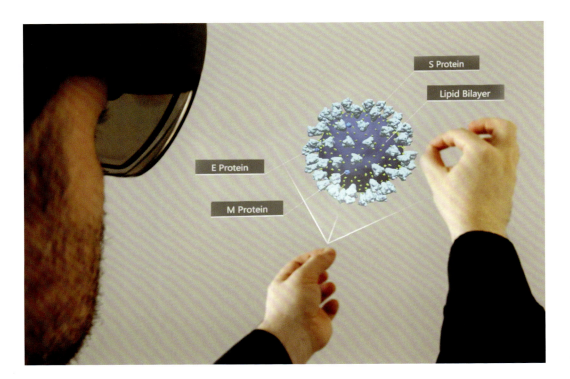

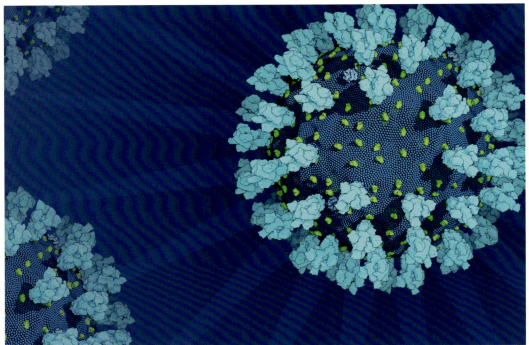

INVIVO – A RED NUCLEUS COMPANY
page 38

invivo.com

The Coronavirus Explorer *(top)*

An interactive HoloLens 2 AR model of the SARS-CoV-2 virus created for anyone who wants to explore its biological structure.

© INVIVO – a Red Nucleus company

COVID-19 and the Science of Soap *(bottom)*

Early in the pandemic, we created this animation to explain the ways soap destroys viruses. The lively neon and toon-shaded style proved popular, leading to multiple translations and a feature on *Forbes*.

© INVIVO – a Red Nucleus company

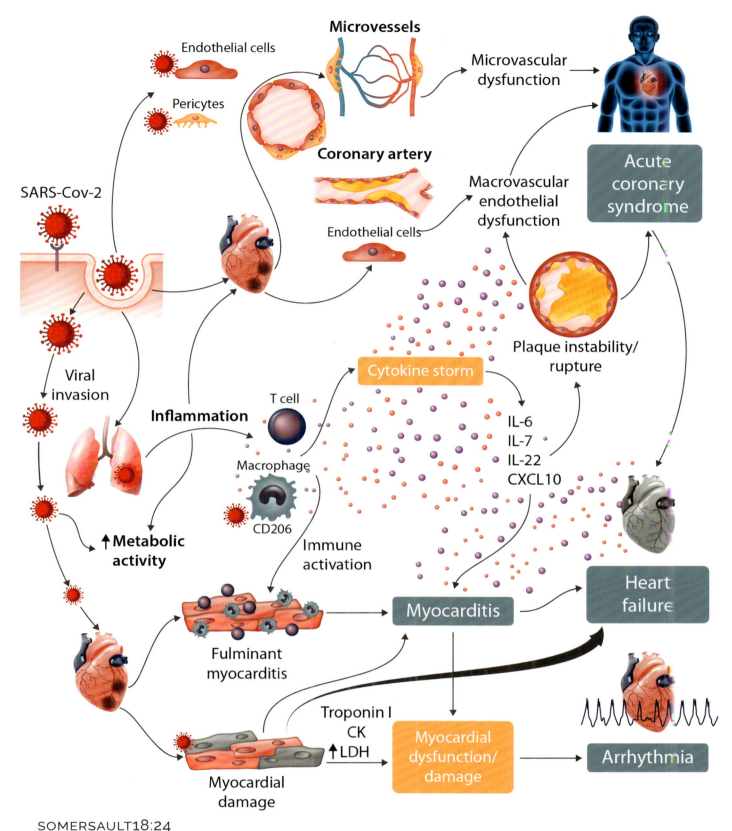

Microvessels

Endothelial cells

Pericytes

Microvascular
dysfunction

Coronary artery

Endothelial cells

SARS-Cov-2

Viral
invasion

Inflammation

↑Metabolic
activity

T cell

Macrophage

CD206

Immune
activation

Cytokine storm

Macrovascular
endothelial
dysfunction

Acute
coronary
syndrome

Plaque instability/
rupture

IL-6
IL-7
IL-22
CXCL10

Fulminant
myocarditis

Myocardial
damage

Troponin I
CK
↑LDH

Myocarditis

Myocardial
dysfunction/
damage

Heart
failure

Arrhythmia

SOMERSAULT18:24

page 141

somersault1824.com

Cardiovascular Involvement in COVID-19

This cover illustration was created for *Cardiovascular Research*, published by Oxford Academic. It shows
the cardiovascular involvement in COVID-19, its key manifestations and hypothetical mechanisms.

Illustration by somersault18:24. © Oxford Academic

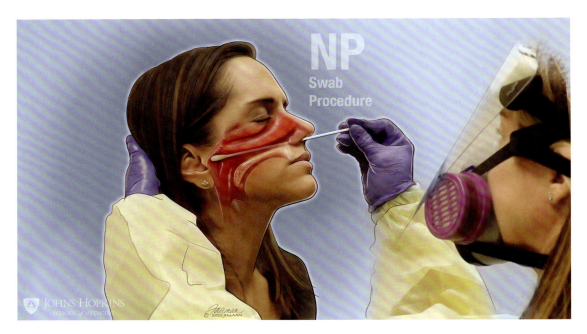

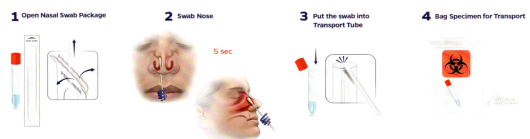

1 Open Nasal Swab Package

2 Swab Nose

5 sec

3 Put the swab into Transport Tube

4 Bag Specimen for Transport

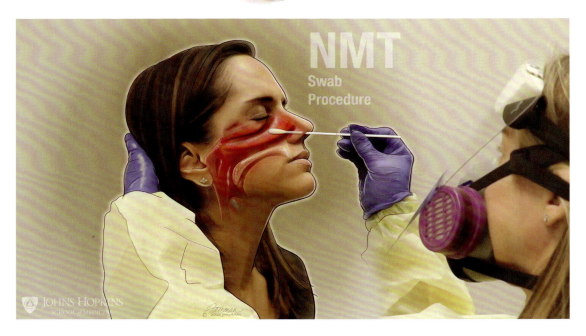

JENNIFER FAIRMAN
page 91

Johns Hopkins University, Dept. of Art As Applied to Medicine
medicalart.johnshopkins.edu/fairman

NP vs. NMT Swabbing Technique

Swabbing procedure for COVID-19 testing.

Illustration: Jennifer E. Fairman, MA, MPS, CMI, FAMI, © 2020, Johns Hopkins University

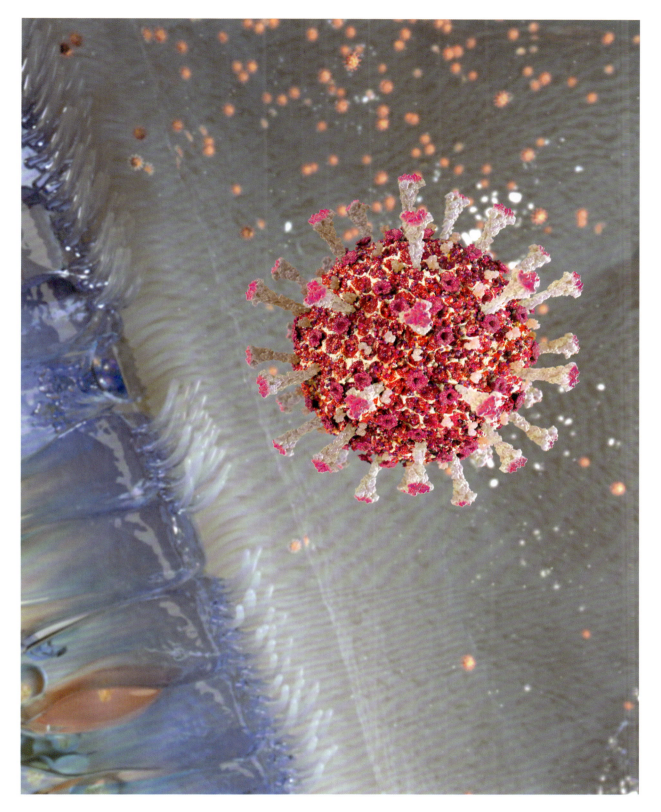

NANBOT MEDICAL SCIENTIFIC COMMUNICATION

page 44

nanobotmedical.com

SARS-CoV-2 Virus Entering a Nasal Cavity

Artistic representation of the SARS-CoV-2 virus.

© Yuriy Svidinenko, Nanobot Medical

Celsion's DNA Vaccine Approach

Polymeric delivery system

Antigen1 DNA sequence
Immune modifier DNA sequence
Antigen 2 DNA sequence

B Cell
BCR
Viral antigen
Muscle Cell

CD8⁺ T Cell
TCR
Viral antigen — CD8
MHC I
Muscle Cell

CD4⁺ T Cell
TCR
Viral antigen — CD4
MHC II
APC

Viral antigen
Viral antigen
MHC I
Viral mRNA
DNA transcription
Nucleus
Proteasome
Muscle Cell

MHC II
Endosome
Lysosome
Viral mRNA
DNA transcription
Nucleus
Proteolytic vesicle
MHC II compartment
Antigen Presenting Cell (APC)

MHC I: Major Histocompatibility Complex class I
MHC II: Major Histocompatibility Complex class II
TCR: T Cell Receptor
BCR: B Cell Receptor
CD4: Cluster of Differentiation 4
CD8: Cluster of Differentiation 8 } Membrane glycoproteins (TCR co-receptors)

JANE WHITNEY

page 152

janewhitney.com

Vaccine Approach
Celsion's next generation vaccine delivers, on a single plasmid, multiple SARS-CoV-2 antigens in conjunction with a potent immune modifier, interleukin-12 (IL-12), which directs a TH-1 immune response.

Illustration by Jane Whitney © Celsion Corporation

SARS-CoV-2 virus
Part of viral RNA that encodes for the spike

Moderna mRNA-1273 vaccine
Nanoliposome containing mRNA:
mRNA, encodes for spike
Lipids
PEG lipids
Cholesterol

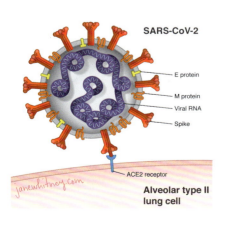

SARS-CoV-2
E protein
M protein
Viral RNA
Spike
ACE2 receptor
Alveolar type II lung cell

(left)
Stylized image of the Sars-CoV-2 virus that causes COVID-19 disease, showing the spike protein and other membrane proteins, as well as the RNA encoding for the virus.

© Jane Whitney

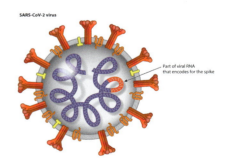

(above)
The Moderna COVID-19 vaccine contains mRNA encoding for the spike protein of the virus, inside a lipid nanoparticle which mimics low-density lipoproteins, and allows them to be taken up by the cells.

© Jane Whitney

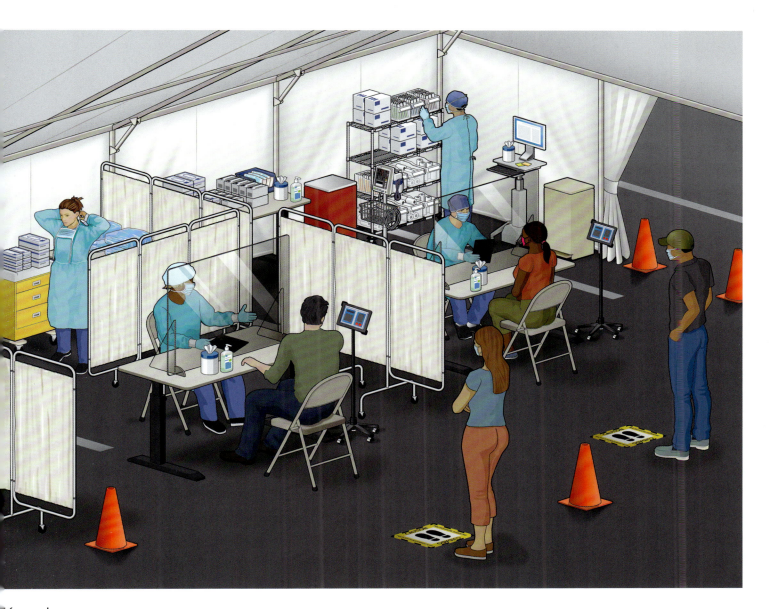

KOPP ILLUSTRATION

page 121

koppillustration.com/medical

This Illustration shows a typical walk-up COIVD-19 testing tent.

© Kopp Illustration

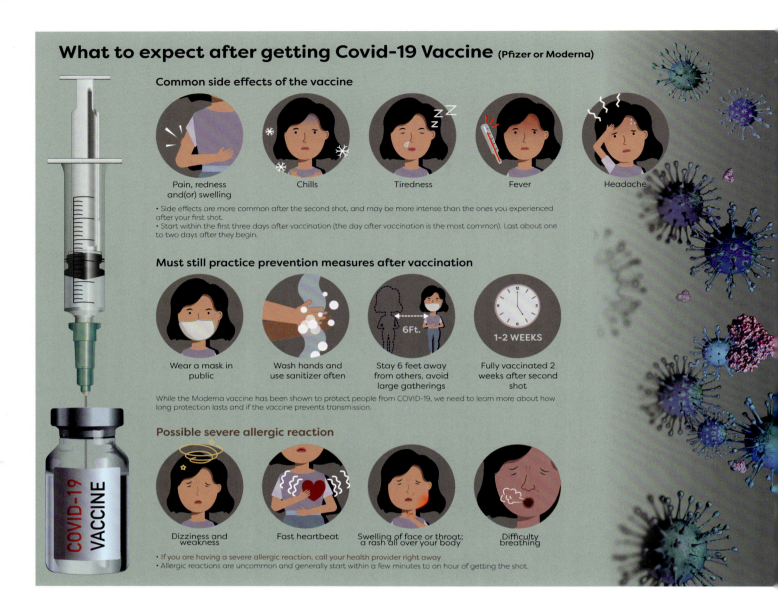

WENRONG HE

page 111

Rochester Institute of Technology
hewena-art.com *

Vaccine Side Effects and Prevention

This digital illustration demonstrates the side effects of the COVID-19 vaccine and prevention measures to take after vaccination. The illustration shows people who need to be vaccinated what to expect after receiving a vaccine.

© Wenrong He

Student Symptom Decision Tree
Screen all students for potential COVID-19 symptoms or exposure

Low-risk: general symptoms

- Fever (≥100.4°F)
- Sore throat
- Congestion/runny nose
- Headache
- Nausea/vomiting/diarrhea
- Fatigue/muscle or body aches

High-risk: red flag symptoms

- **Cough**
- **Difficulty breathing**
- **Loss of taste/smell**

Exposure to COVID-19 positive person? *Close contact: Within 6 ft for > 15 minutes cumulative (regardless of mask)*

NO

▸ 1 **low risk** symptom → STOP → Send home → Return to school 24 hrs after symptom resolution (without fever reducing medication)

▸ ≥2 **low risk** symptoms OR 1 **high risk** symptom → STOP → Send home → Evaluation by health care provider

1. Health care provider confirms alternative diagnosis for symptoms. A health care provider's note must be on file. SARS-CoV-2 PCR test not needed. → Return to school after 24 hrs without fever and symptoms improving

2. **Negative** SARS-CoV-2 PCR test. → Return to school after 24 hrs without fever and symptoms improving

3. **Positive** SARS-CoV-2 PCR test OR No provider visit or test. → **Return to school only after 10 days since symptom onset and 24 hrs without fever. Quarantine close contacts of confirmed cases. Contact HCA if questions.**

YES → STOP → Stay home* → **Return to school after 10 days from last exposure, unless symptoms develop. Continue symptom monitoring through 14 days after last exposure. If symptoms develop obtain a PCR test.**

*In consultation with OC Health Care Agency (HCA)

OC health CARE AGENCY

This care pathway was designed to assist school personnel and is not intended to replace the clinician's judgment or establish a protocol for all patients with a particular condition. Diagnosis and treatment should be under the close supervision of a qualified health care provider. Guidance might change 12-10-2020

SOMERSAULT18:24

page 141

somersault1824.com

COVID-19 Student Symptom Decision Tree for the Orange County Health Care Agency

A Decision Tree showing measures to be followed when a student shows symptoms, has close contact or is confirmed positive with COVID-19.

Orange County Healthcare Agency. Illustration by somersault18:24.

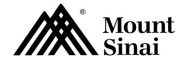

COVID-19

I have:

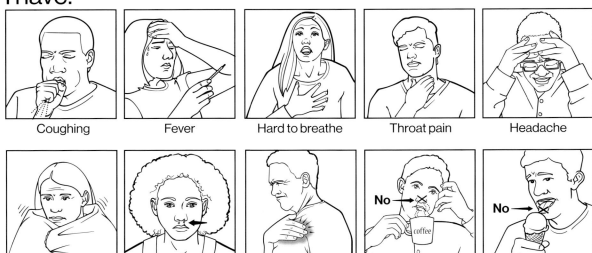

| Coughing | Fever | Hard to breathe | Throat pain | Headache |

| Chills / shaking | Runny nose | Muscle pain | Problem with smell | Problem with taste |

How many days sick?

Month

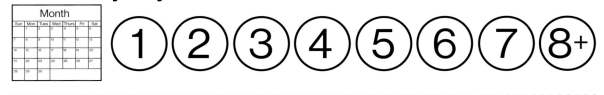

(1) (2) (3) (4) (5) (6) (7) (8+)

Me

Yes
No

Interpreter needed?

Yes
No

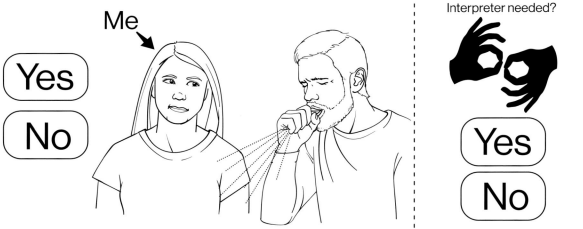

Created by Jill K. Gregory, Instructional Technology Group | April 2020 | ©2020 Mount Sinai Health System

JILL GREGORY

Icahn School of Medicine at Mount Sinai
www.jillkgregory.com

A COVID-19 screening tool used for patients who are Hard of Hearing or Deaf. The written language and content were created in consultation with Interpretive Services and Patient Education..

Jill Gregory ©2020 Mount Sinai Health System

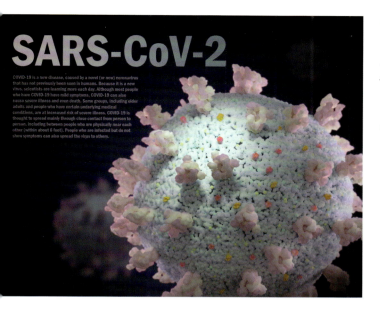

SangEun Cha

Joonhoe Kim
joonhoekim.wixsite.com/jkim

3D reconstruction of SARS-CoV-2

© SangEun Cha, Joonhoe Kim

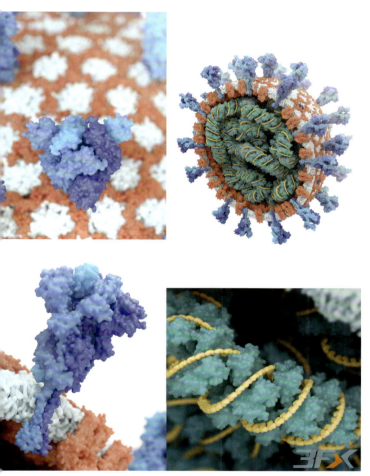

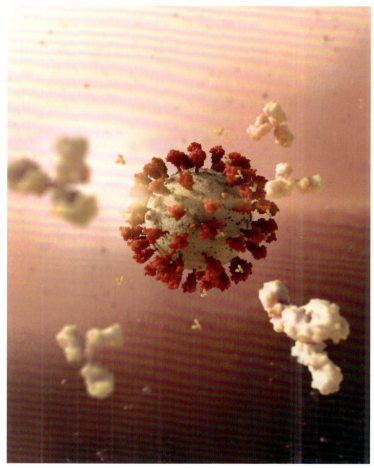

3FX, INC.

age 10-11

fx.com

1 2020, everyone in the world was frightened by a strange new virus that ad taken over. Our thought as medical animators was that SARS-CoV-2 night not be so scary if we could just see what it looked like.

) 3fx, Inc.

LampScience

page 39

lampscience.com

Immune System Response to Sars-CoV-2

Since SARS-CoV-2 is a new emergent virus, there is no pre-existing immunity, and the whole of humanity is susceptible to infection and the development of COVID-19 disease.

© LampScience

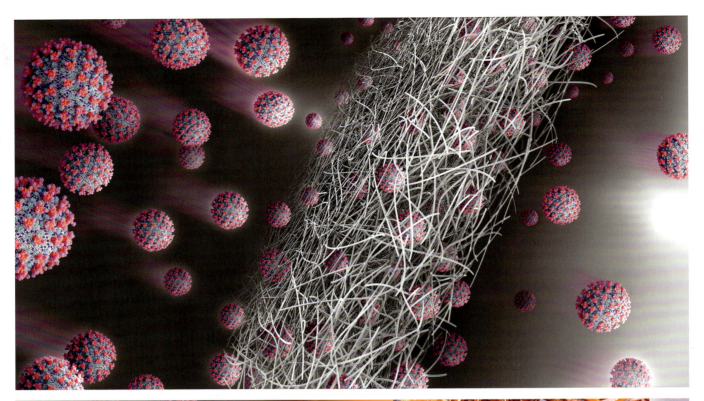

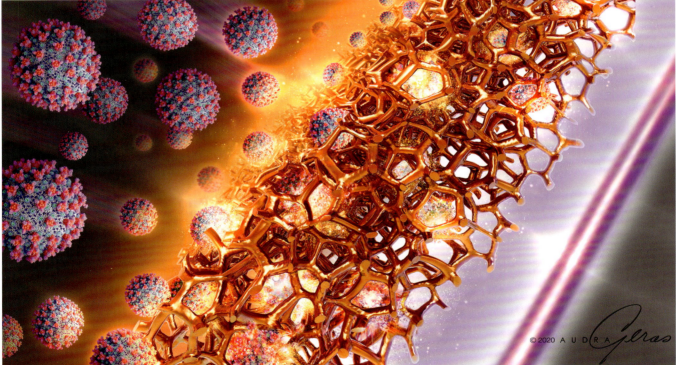

AUDRA GERAS

page 30-31

Geras Healthcare Productions

audrageras.com

HVAC Filtration Comparison

This image depicts a comparison in the efficiency of standard HVAC filtration versus that of a novel heated nickel filtration technology in the elimination of COVID-19 from circulated air.

© 2020 Audra Geras

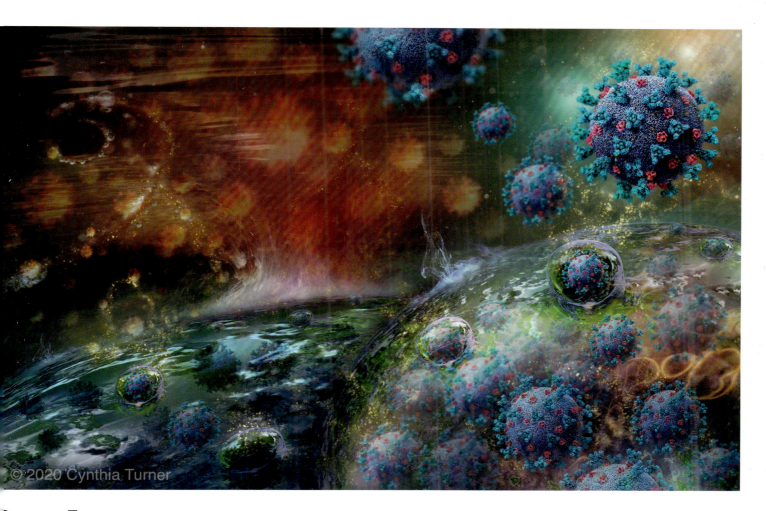

© 2020 Cynthia Turner

CYNTHIA TURNER

age 52-53

lexander & Turner Inc. Medical Illustration Studio

lexanderandturner.com

ytokine Storm

iral budding from the plasma membrane of lung epithelial cells enables coronaviruses to exit the ost cell after infection and replication. This can initiate a cytokine storm, a sudden over-response f the body's immune system all at once from an immune system gone awry, producing an flammatory response flaring out of control.

2020 Cynthia Turner

I CAN REMEMBER LISTENING TO THE TV EARLY IN THE MORNING ON SEPTEMBER 11TH, 2001. WE ALL KNOW WHAT HAPPENED: THE CHAOS, THE QUESTIONS, THE SURPRISE AND THE UNKNOWN FUTURE TO COME. BACK THEN, I WAS RUNNING MY SMALL STUDIO PRACTICE OUT OF RENTED OFFICE SPACE WHICH WAS WALKING DISTANCE FROM MY APARTMENT. I DIDN'T KNOW THE FULL IMPACT OF WHAT WAS HAPPENING IN THAT MOMENT. WITH PROJECTS ON MY MIND, I TURNED THE TV OFF TOO SOON AND WAS FOCUSED ON GETTING TO WORK EARLY IN A HURRY.

WHEN I GOT THERE, I TURNED THE RADIO ON TO NPR. THAT'S WHEN REALITY BEGAN TO SINK IN. I SAT FOCUSED ON IMPENDING DEADLINES, BUT SUDDENLY REALIZED THAT NONE OF IT MATTERED. HUNDREDS OF PEOPLE WERE DYING AS I SAT THERE. IN THAT INSTANT, MY ROLE AS A MEDICAL ILLUSTRATOR WAS COMPLETELY IRRELEVANT. DEEP SHAME CAME OVER ME. I FELT COMPLETELY WORTHLESS TO THOSE WHO WERE SUFFERING AT THAT MOMENT.

"I AM JUST A USELESS ARTIST. HOW CAN I HELP?" I DON'T THINK ANYONE ENTERS OUR PROFESSION EVER THINKING THAT THEY MIGHT FEEL THAT WAY ABOUT THEIR CHOICE TO BECOME A SCIENCE COMMUNICATOR. THERE WAS A TIME MUCH EARLIER THAN COLLEGE THAT I ASPIRED TO BECOME A PEDIATRICIAN, A USEFUL HEALTH PROFESSIONAL. ON 9-11, I FELT HELPLESS AND DEEP REGRET THAT I HAD MADE THE WRONG CHOICE.

THOUGH THE US WAS EXPERIENCING A TARGETED CRISIS, THE ENTIRE WORLD FELT IT. PEOPLE CAME TOGETHER, PUT ASIDE THEIR DIFFERENCES AND HELPED IN EVERY WAY POSSIBLE. STRANGERS GREETED EACH OTHER WITH EXTRA KINDNESS AS MANY FELT ISOLATED AND HELPLESS. THIS WAS WHAT WOULD BECOME ONE OF THOSE TIMES THE WORLD CAME TOGETHER TO FIGHT AN ELUSIVE KILLER.

NOW WE ARE FACING A SIMILAR MOMENT. WHEN THE FIRST MURMURS HIT THE MEDIA THAT A NOVEL CORONAVIRUS HAD BEEN DISCOVERED IN AN OPEN MARKET IN WUHAN, A CITY IN CHINA'S HUBEI PROVINCE, WE KNEW WE MIGHT BE FACING YET ANOTHER ELUSIVE KILLER. THE QUESTIONS BEGAN TO FLOOD: WHO IS PATIENT ZERO? WHAT HOST DID IT ORIGINATE FROM? HOW FAST DOES THE VIRUS MUTATE? HOW DOES IT COMPARE TO THE COMMON FLU? WHAT ARE THE BEST WAYS TO PREVENT THE SPREAD? WHAT MAKES ONE PATIENT MORE SUSCEPTIBLE THAN ANOTHER? WAS IT CARRIED INTO THE MARKET FROM A NEARBY FARM? WILL WE EVER DEVELOP AN EFFECTIVE VACCINE? WHEN WILL THE WORLD GO BACK TO NORMAL? WITH A BOUNDLESS GLOBAL ECONOMY, IT INEVITABLY WOULD MAKE ITS WAY INTO EVERYONE'S BACKYARD IN A MATTER OF TIME.

EPIDEMIC BECAME PANDEMIC. MORTALITY CONTINUES AS I WRITE AND AS RESEARCHERS FRANTICALLY WORK TO FIND ANSWERS, EFFECTIVE TREATMENTS, AND A CURE. OUR FIELD IS SEEING A SURGE WHERE WE CAN'T DRAW PICTURES FAST ENOUGH: INDEED, THERE HAVE BEEN SO MANY THAT I HAVE LOST COUNT! OUR BEST WEAPON IS RAPID, WIDE-SPREAD, EFFECTIVE COMMUNICATION OF TRUSTED FACTUAL INFORMATION AND THE DISCREDITING POLARIZED AND POLITICIZED MISINFORMATION IN A FRAGMENTED MEDIA ENVIRONMENT.

THE WORLD IS IN CRISIS AGAIN WITH ONE MAJOR DIFFERENCE:
I AM NEEDED. WE ARE NEEDED.

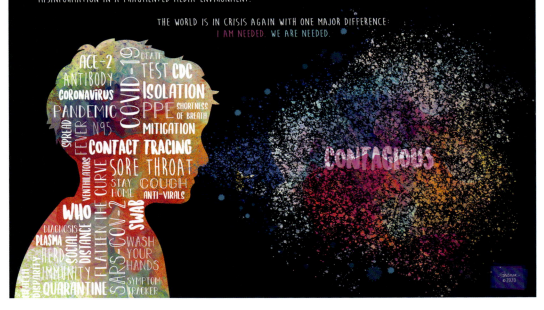

JENNIFER FAIRMAN

page 91

Fairman Studios, LLC / Illustr8.Science
fairmanstudios.com

A Big Sneeze: COVID Colloquialism

The virus has had an immeasurable impact on so many facets of our lives, both professionally and personally. This was a personal piece I created as I was contemplating what a full year of quarantining while fighting a virus with visual information has meant to me as a medical illustrator. This piece represents my absorbing and making sense of what I call "COVID Colloquialism" and the new vocabulary that has pervaded every conversation I have had regarding the pandemic. It's just a big sneeze of information overload.

Illustration: Jennifer E. Fairman, MA, MPS, CMI, FAMI, © 2020, Fairman Studios